W9-ARH-829

Welcome to the **EVERYTHING**® series!

These handy, accessible books give you all you need to tackle a difficult project, gain a new hobby, comprehend a fascinating topic, prepare for an exam, or even brush up on something you learned back in school but have since forgotten.

You can read an *EVERYTHING*® book from cover-to-cover or just pick out the information you want from our four useful boxes: e-facts, e-ssentials, e-alerts, and e-questions. We literally give you everything you need to know on the subject, but throw in a lot of fun stuff along the way, too.

We now have well over 100 *EVERYTHING*® books in print, spanning such wide-ranging topics as weddings, pregnancy, wine, learning guitar, one-pot cooking, managing people, and so much more. When you're done reading them all, you can finally say you know *EVERYTHING*®!

E FACTS
Important sound bytes of information

E SSENTIALS
Quick handy tips

E ALERT
Urgent warnings

E QUESTIONS?
Solutions to common problems

THE EVERYTHING Series

Dear Reader,

While writing this book, I tried hard to keep in mind what you may already know and may want to know about T'ai Chi and QiGong. Because we haven't met and I don't know exactly what drew you to being curious enough about T'ai Chi and QiGong to pick up the book, I covered the subject from many different vantage points. The writing was fun and confirmed my deepest feeling about these two remarkable activities: The range of T'ai Chi and QiGong is astonishing. Only something so ancient, something that has been created by so many disciplined and highly skilled people and from a remarkable culture could offer so much in such a simple form.

If beauty is in the eye of the beholder, I believe that T'ai Chi and QiGong have taught me how to behold the beauty of life where I would have otherwise missed it. In Western culture, which is devoted to youth as the best life has to offer, T'ai Chi and QiGong have taught me the wonder of maturing. In a life filled with joys, simple pleasures, irritations, and tragedy, they have taught me how to find acceptance and inner peace with life as it is. T'ai Chi and QiGong have given me the tools to direct my awareness into parts of my body that have been sick, and to return to health more quickly. I have found a world of life's beauty and personal health available through it, and I hope you do, too.

Sincerely,

Ellae Elinwood

THE
EVERYTHING®
T'AI CHI AND QIGONG BOOK

Enjoy good health, longevity,
and a stress-free life

Ellae Elinwood

3 1571 00206 9162

GLEN COVE PUBLIC LIBRARY
4 GLEN COVE AVENUE
GLEN COVE, NEW YORK 11542-2885

Adams Media Corporation
Avon, Massachusetts

To Dotty Campbell, my mom, who taught me the T'ai Chi of life.

• • •

EDITORIAL
Publishing Director: Gary M. Krebs
Managing Editor: Kate McBride
Copy Chief: Laura MacLaughlin
Acquisitions Editor: Allison Carpenter Yoder
Development Editors: Tere Drenth,
        Lesley Bolton,
        Michael Paydos

PRODUCTION
Production Director: Susan Beale
Production Manager: Michelle Roy Kelly
Series Designer: Daria Perreault
Layout and Graphics: Arlene Apone,
Paul Beatrice, Brooke Camfield,
Colleen Cunningham, Daria Perreault,
Frank Rivera

Copyright ©2002, Adams Media Corporation.
All rights reserved. This book, or parts thereof, may not be reproduced
in any form without permission from the publisher; exceptions
are made for brief excerpts used in published reviews.

An Everything® Series Book.
Everything® is a registered trademark of Adams Media Corporation.

Published by Adams Media Corporation
57 Littlefield Street, Avon, MA 02322 U.S.A.
www.adamsmedia.com

ISBN: 1-58062-646-7
Printed in the United States of America.

J I H G F E D C B A

Library of Congress Cataloging-in-Publication Data available from publisher.

This publication is designed to provide accurate and authoritative information with regard to the subject matter covered. It is sold with the understanding that the publisher is not engaged in rendering legal, accounting, or other professional advice. If legal advice or other expert assistance is required, the services of a competent professional person should be sought.
    —From a *Declaration of Principles* jointly adopted by a Committee of the American Bar Association and a Committee of Publishers and Associations

Illustrations by Barry Littmann.
Photographs courtesy of Robert Frost.

This book is available at quantity discounts for bulk purchases.
For information, call 1-800-872-5627.

Visit the entire Everything® series at everything.com

Contents

Introduction

Welcome to the exercise phenomenon of the millennium: T'ai Chi and QiGong. T'ai Chi is a movement activity, while QiGong is an ancient form of breathing skills. The two in tandem can bring you better health, a better shot at longevity, and a wonderful sense of inner peace.

These simple, flowing activities have gone from being almost unknown in the Western world in the 1950s to having a worldwide following of hundreds of thousands of people today. T'ai Chi and QiGong are practiced by stressed businesspeople, overworked parents, media and TV stars, musicians, politicians, and you!

Over the last fifty years, people have shown an increasing interest in blending and balancing the wisdom of the ancient East with the technology of the modern Western world, and T'ai Chi and QiGong are perfect examples of the success of this combination. T'ai Chi and QiGong are thousands of years old and over the centuries they have been honed by each person who has mastered them and passed their knowledge along. Now those who practice T'ai Chi and QiGong in the West have found improved balance, reduced stress, and help in recovering from surgery and injuries, to name just a few benefits. T'ai Chi and QiGong can contribute greatly to your physical, mental, emotional, and spiritual well-being.

One addition benefit of T'ai Chi and QiGong is that, just like the best things in life, it's free. You don't need an expensive gym, expensive clothes or equipment, or special requirements—you can focus on just you and these lovely ancient activities. The cost to learn T'ai Chi and QiGong is minimal (not usually free, but close).

Another plus is that because T'ai Chi and QiGong involve gentle, non-forceful movements, you won't have to pay expensive medical bills recovering from sustained injuries.

In this book, then, you'll discover the wonderful benefits of T'ai Chi and QiGong, demonstrated in fantastic photos. You'll also find fun and useful sidebars, stories, and tips. And at the end of the book, you'll find a list of sources for books, videos, seminars, summer camps, magazines, and Internet Web sites to further your experience.

I hope you enjoy your journey of discovering for yourself these wonderful gifts from ancient China.

CHAPTER 1

Understanding T'ai Chi and QiGong

T'ai Chi is a nearly perfect form of exercise for anyone—from athletes to people not able to walk. For any stage of life and health, T'ai Chi can work wonders. The breathing activity of QiGong was designed to draw in, fill up on, and then deliberately cultivate one's chi, or vital force. By using these methods, you can take charge of your mental, physical, emotional, and spiritual well-being.

What Is T'ai Chi?

T'ai Chi (pronounced TIE CHEE and sometimes spelled Taiji) involves a series of prescribed positions done in predictable, flowing sequences that use every muscle and joint in the body. These sequences are slow, relaxed, stylized, comfortable motions that look a bit like swimming without the water. So T'ai Chi is a series of positions, one flowing into the next. By gently twisting and turning as you balance and rebalance your arms and legs in a lovely, unhurried, steady, graceful sequence, every portion of the body is used, refreshed, and revitalized.

ESSENTIALS

T'ai Chi and QiGong both support any physical activity you may do. Because of the very nature of these ancient flowing and freeing motions, they can enhance any other activity you're doing. And while T'ai Chi and QiGong balance each other, they can also be done separately with satisfying results.

If you're seeing T'ai Chi practiced for the first time, what likely catches your attention is the grace, poise, and serenity emanating from the practitioner. That is how T'ai Chi looks from the outside. To the person doing the movements, it is a calming, centering, quieting experience that improves your feeling of personal well-being and general health.

In addition, doctors find that the practice improves a variety of patients' nagging health issues. Spiritual teachers find that it encourages a state of mind that facilitates spiritual development in any faith. School teachers see that it enhances the focus and concentration of students.

What Does T'ai Chi Ch'uan Mean?

The words T'ai Chi Ch'uan are pronounced TIE CHEE CHEWAN, and, like much of Chinese, are not easy to put into a simple translation. The words T'ai Chi Ch'uan are from the *I Ching*, the Chinese Book of Changes, which embodies the Chinese philosophy and faith of Taoism. (The Taoist philosophy was expressed by famed Chinese philosopher Lao

Tzu in his book the *Tao Te Ching*.) T'ai Chi means "supreme ultimate": In the beginning of all things, there is oneness, and then the oneness divides into two forces—the female force of yin and the male force of yang. In the nanosecond of the division is where T'ai Chi is. Ch'uan, on the other hand, means "fisted hand." So T'ai Chi Ch'uan means "supreme ultimate fisted hand."

T'ai Chi Ch'uan was developed by the ancient Chinese monk/warriors as a martial art. In that time, many monks' spiritual development was combined with the warrior's path. The goal was to have a peaceful inner world connected to the oneness of life and also to put tremendous martial art skills into action. The perfection was to be able to maintain peace and warrior skills at the same time, at any time.

The practice began somewhere between 550 B.C. to A.D. 1300. T'ai Chi Ch'uan was taught and transmitted through the centuries in secrecy. The teaching was passed from master to student in the strictest of privacy. For centuries, the secrets of T'ai Chi Ch'uan were well guarded among a privileged few, but in the 1800s, the practice was exposed to the Chinese general public, and later to the West.

How Is T'ai Chi Different from Other Forms of Exercise?

The roots of the beginning of T'ai Chi Ch'uan (the "Ch'uan" has today been dropped because the "fist" portion of the term is rarely the focus) marks it immediately as unique. It was developed with the express purpose of providing an embodied experience of oneness with all things, and then applying that wisdom to a disciplined and competitive form of martial arts. Through movement, T'ai Chi fills the practitioner with *chi*, the Chinese word for "life force" or "energy." This chi—and the mastery of and mental directing of chi—that comes from T'ai Chi positions as you flow from one position to another, marks T'ai Chi Ch'uan as completely unique. In other words, no other form of activity so successfully combines health, well-being, and vitality in lovely, graceful movements that remind all parts of the body, mind, and spirit to open and coordinate with one another.

FACTS

- **T'ai Chi:** Supreme ultimate
- **T'ai Chi Ch'uan:** Supreme ultimate fist
- **Chi:** The cosmic energy flow of life
- **QiGong** (also spelled Ch'i Kung): The use of breathing to develop the chi for special purposes, such as fighting and healing
- **T'ai Chi Master:** A highly skilled teacher of T'ai Chi
- **Tan t'ien:** Deep in the center of the belly one and one-third inches below the navel—a place for centering yourself and a gathering place for chi

Who Uses T'ai Chi?

Gyms worldwide abound with folks lifting weights for health. Roads and paths teem with runners, walkers, and bikers exercising for fun, pleasure, and health. Mountains provide playgrounds for snowboarding, skiing, and the like. Endorphins released into the body through these activities create a wonderful feeling of well-being.

People engage in all forms of physical activity engaged for many reasons. Yet only Eastern disciplines—T'ai Chi and QiGong in this case—provide the benefits of other activities in just a half-hour of practice each day. As a result of these varied and valuable benefits, T'ai Chi is done by the famous, the unknown, the flamboyant, those who live simply, the proud, and the humble. All ethnicities, creeds, and income/social status use T'ai Chi. It knows no boundaries between people, teaches equality and simplicity of heart and mind, and has great and lasting benefits for one and all.

Several forms of T'ai Chi are taught throughout the world. For a long time, these forms could be learned only from a specific teacher. Now, with videos, television, the Internet, and books and magazines, instruction is much easier to come by. You can find an array of T'ai Chi forms being offered, but the most common T'ai Chi form now taught is the Yang method. (This book teaches the Yang method.) Start with this form and then if you decide to learn another, you will see that although the forms are different, they enhance each other. See the "Which T'ai Chi Method

Is Best for You?" section, later in this chapter, for more information on T'ai Chi methods.

Why Take the Time to Learn T'ai Chi?

T'ai Chi isn't really exercise as we know it. It doesn't rely on anything besides you and your body to make it possible, so one reason to learn it is convenience. You can do the practice anywhere, at any time, while dressed in anything. The limits are only what seem appropriate to you. Another reason to learn T'ai Chi is that it requires no extra props. You don't need a gym. You don't need special shoes. You don't need a road, path, or trail. You don't need special clothes, gear, or expensive tickets to anywhere to enjoy it. You need only your positions, a bit of space, and some air to breathe. That's it. These flowing movements contribute to so many aspects of better health that the benefits quickly become clear. You can feel greater vitality and youthfulness in a very few weeks of dedicated learning.

ESSENTIALS

T'ai Chi's philosophy can be taken up at any life stage or situation. You don't need to become stronger, improve your flexibility, drop some weight, or improve your health before you can start. You can start right now. Even if you have only partial movement, move what you can. Let it work for you now, as you are.

Take a deep and easy breath right now. Don't move or change in any way, just breathe. Now breathe again. Move or adjust how you're sitting or standing if you need to. Now breathe again. Do you notice how this simple exercise requires no previous experience or level of fitness? So it is with T'ai Chi (and QiGong, too).

Anyone who is drawn to T'ai Chi can learn and benefit from it. You can learn it from a book, from a video, or with an instructor. Although T'ai Chi is usually shown as a standing activity, it is also possible to modify the motions for anyone who has a limited range of movement (see Chapter 12). A friend of mine started QiGong in bed and as she healed from her accident, she progressed to a seated T'ai Chi until she was able to stand comfortably and do both QiGong and

T'ai Chi standing. Even folks who are confined to a chair or bed can adapt movements from the sequences and improve range of motion, joint suppleness, and breathing ability. I taught a form of T'ai Chi in convalescent hospitals in the 1970s, altering the practice to be accessible to the lovely elderly people confined to their chairs. It was a popular class and the breathing and movement helped each participant each time he or she did it.

This doesn't mean that T'ai Chi (or QiGong) is limited to a time when you are elderly or unable to stand—not at all! T'ai Chi is practiced by superb athletes as well. T'ai Chi is a unique activity in that it can be used beneficially in so many walks of life.

You'll know you've begun to master T'ai Chi by the predictable sequence of movements. You'll know one posture as it flows into the next. You will be feeling quieter in your mind and more balanced and graceful in your walking and moving. Your breathing will be more relaxed and more open. You will no longer wonder whether you have it right or what foot you should have your weight on now.

You may also feel that although you've learned the basic postures and movements, like reading a great book you can tell there is more good stuff ahead. You'll be ready for the next step—continuing your practice and relaxing into it.

What Is the Cost?

Because no special equipment is required and the information about the sequenced motions is readily available, there is precious little required to start. Your only expense will for the method of instruction you choose: a video (about $30), a private class (about $40), or a group class (about $10). Of course, you can make it as expensive as you choose with special (but not truly necessary) clothes and shoes, trips to T'ai Chi intensives and camps, and subscriptions to magazines and book clubs. But these are all extras and even though they add variety and enhance learning, they are not in the least essential for the initial learning and practice of your own T'ai Chi activity.

Which T'ai Chi Method Is Best?

T'ai Chi has evolved over time into schools of practice. Two such schools are Wu and Yang. Both are excellent forms to benefit from T'ai Chi. The Wu includes small moves and a body technique designed for combat. The Yang emphasizes graceful movements for health.

In this book, you will learn the Yang form—the most common form of T'ai Chi currently being taught in the Western world. You will have an easier time moving from this book into another book, a video, or instruction if you're learning a form that is commonly taught. The Yang method is also the form of T'ai Chi most associated with health, inner peace, and well-being.

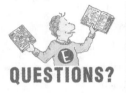

QUESTIONS?

What does T'ai Chi have to do with martial arts?
Martial arts in the ancient world didn't simply mean self-defense, but a way of life for its practitioners, who became both monks and warriors, the revered balance of Old China.

T'ai Chi without the Ch'uan is enjoyed by many as a tool for better health, longevity, and improved well-being.

QiGong—Developing the Internal Force

The older spelling of QiGong is Chi-Kung and is pronounced CHEE GONG. Chi means the complete and vital life force that brings life to all things. Kung means the correct way. Chi-Kung (now QiGong), then, means the correct way to have complete and vital life force. Chi has also been translated as "energy" and kung as "exercise," so another meaning is "energy exercise." In the Western world, this art of breathing has been transmitted under a different spelling, QiGong, which is pronounced KEY GONG. Both QiGong and Chi-Kung mean the same thing, so whether you take a class in QiGong or a class in Chi-Kung, you'll be learning basically the same breathing art.

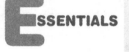

ESSENTIALS Because Chinese is such a varied language, translations also vary. QiGong and Chi-Kung have been translated as the following: "breath skill," "the use of the breathing to develop," and "the art of energy."

How Can QiGong Help?

This book focuses on the health aspects of QiGong. These breathing practices, then, can be used to prepare for or support your T'ai Chi exercises. (Some T'ai Chi teachers recommend learning QiGong before you learn T'ai Chi.) Or you can do them separately.

The five branches of QiGong all share the common theme of rooting the body through correct breathing to increase and focus the circulation of the chi. In successfully rooting the chi in the body, the first step toward inner force and vital health is attained. Each of these five branches uses slightly different methods and practices, but the goal is the same: inner calm, inner force, and inner vitality. Under this umbrella word of QiGong are breath-training systems that cultivate cosmic or vital energy. The effects on the body, mind, and spirit as a result of the QiGong practice are rich and varied. Learning QiGong provides a support for so many aspects of your life—health, mind expansion and focus, spiritual cultivation, and combat effectiveness are a few.

How Does QiGong Work?

Breath is the first and most important life-giving force for your body. You can go for many days without food, many hours without water, but only a very few minutes without air. Health attitudes of the ancient Chinese acknowledged not only that to be vital the body must breathe, but also acknowledged the more subtle aspects of what breathing could achieve.

Air is composed of gases—primarily oxygen. The ancient Chinese believed the air to be filled with vital life force necessary to all living things. This great, vital, animating force of life was called chi. Chi was seen as not only desirable, but also necessary, to draw in, fill up, and store.

Without chi taken in through the breath, there is no life. Without movement of the body, breathing cannot be deep or fulfilling. In order for the body to reach better and better levels of health, the first step needs to be chi-enhanced breathing combined with body movement to enhance the blood, bones, muscles, and skin. The breath draws in the chi, and the movement disperses it throughout the body: Vitality and energy result. This cultivation of the chi to benefit the body, mind, and spirit is the very foundation of all Chinese health and martial arts.

When chi is able to circulate throughout the body unhindered, the body perceptions and feelings become clearer (not more powerful, but clearer). The muscles become more filled with vitality, and your sense of touch becomes more alert. When you attain this state of balance and alert aliveness, the moods of anger, depression, and fear tend to become part of the balance. They don't go away—they just become part of the fabric of emotional life. They don't loom larger than the rest, but are more easily accessed at the right time, in the appropriate amount, and then they can be reduced back into the balanced emotional life.

FACTS

When a person becomes angry, the chi becomes coarse and harsh. When the chi is harsh, the feet lose their ground and the personal inner power of harmony is lost. When QiGong is practiced, however, the chi is peaceful and clear. When the chi is peaceful and clear, it is harmonious—just as you are in your inner world.

Chinese medicine is based on the idea that we are each a living system interconnected to the whole of life. All of life (liveliness) comes from chi. The Chinese further believe in many different kinds of energy (or chi), in the universe and when these kinds of energies flow through us, giving life and liveliness to our bodies, they are the reason life exists within us. These different kinds of energies are connected to our body's organs flowing on little highways of chi called meridians that circulate throughout everyone's body.

There are said to be twelve meridians, each nourishing a specific organ. Each different kind of chi that flows, riverlike, through each meridian also affects everything in the person that matches that particular chi characteristic. This has an enormous effect on the person. Moods, taste in foods, inclination toward healthy balance, or how that balance may go off into illness are all profoundly influenced by these chi flows. As the meridians pass through arms, legs, head, and torso in a continuous flow of chi, these all-important meridians can be stimulated or calmed down as needed for a healthy balance by QiGong practices. These routes of chi coursing through the body carry all the life-enhancing properties attributed to QiGong. QiGong is the tool to get them to work at maximum benefit for you. It is the chi that brings enhancement, and QiGong is the cultivator.

Vital force is the bottom line in all health and well-being in the body, mind, and spirit. QiGong, then, becomes the first and most important step before anything else in the living system of a person can be improved.

FACTS

The tan t'ien is located one and one-third inches, or two finger widths, below the navel, buried deep inside the pelvis. It is the center of awareness or energy that you focus on as you do your breathing exercises. The tan t'ien is seen as an all-important storage vessel for chi. When this center is full, your life force is high and healthy. When it is depleted from lack of attention, poor health and lack of well-being manifest in the body.

What Is the Correct Way to Breathe?

Note how a child breathes. It is not high in the chest, but low in the abdomen. Children don't usually have a lot of history with misfortune or accidents, so they approach an experience with their breath deep and open, constrict the breath during an accident, and return to open breath after the accident is over. As young children, we were more present in life—more open to it. It is after we get a series of memories around misfortunes that we shorten our breath, not just before an accident occurs, but all the time. The fear of uncertainty in life events—a fear that is often justifiable—alters our breathing and our ability to cultivate chi.

It doesn't take many years beyond early childhood before we have deeply restricted our breath. Constricted breathing is when, for example, we breathe only into the upper chest. Through limited breathing, we are in a state of limited oxygen, reduced chi, and, therefore, a reduced sense of well-being or more stress (just what you need!). When something unexpected happens, we feel even greater stress. This often makes the situation we're responding to worse than it is. It certainly hampers our ability to respond in a calm, well-thought-out manner.

The goal in QiGong is to breathe through all of life's vagaries like a child who has no fear of something before it occurs and easily readjusts his or her breathing afterwards. Become accustomed to correct breathing, low in the abdomen. By doing QiGong on a regular basis, you remind your body of how to breathe for health of your body, mind, and spirit.

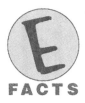

FACTS

The breathing principles of QiGong can be summed up as follows:

- **Natural breath:** The regular breath you take constantly without awareness.
- **Cleansing breath:** Inhaling through the nose and exhaling through the mouth.
- **Tonic breath:** Inhaling through the mouth and exhaling through the nose.
- **Alternate breath:** Inhaling through one nostril, exhaling through the other.
- **Natural, deep breath:** A natural, deep breath taken spontaneously.
- **Long breath:** Abdominal breathing.
- **Reverse long breath:** The abdomen expands when exhaling and contracts when inhaling.
- **Tortoise breath:** Mastery breathing—slow breathing that occurs naturally in masters, often after decades of daily practice.

How Can QiGong Help Today?

Judging from the length of time QiGong has been around—at least 3,000 years—I think I can safely say that this simple, graceful, and powerful breathing skill enhanced the lives of ancient practitioners so much that they passed the tradition of QiGong along. The Chinese have a long history of adding to and honing their exercise arts until they become extremely effective. QiGong benefited these ancients so satisfyingly that they continued to improve it further.

Very little has changed in human bodies over the last few thousand years. Any benefit that QiGong extended to the ancient Chinese is still available to us today. We may actually need it more now for reasons that didn't exist in the ancient world: the lower air quality and our lack of constant and consistent exercise. Our bodies are often doing one thing—sitting, for example—and our minds are doing something very different—working with a computer. These elements of modern life create a compromised daily environment for our bodies. And because the health of our bodies is so fundamental to the functioning of the mind and spirit, QiGong's wisdom brings a badly needed source of health for body, mind, and spirit. Breathing with your QiGong exercises can promote a feeling of well-being and pleasure through the simple act of moving, making breathing and exercising in unison a more natural, desired part of your day. (And if your air quality is bad, do the exercises when your air is the clearest: early morning, perhaps, or in front of an air purifier.)

In the practice of T'ai Chi, some teachers sometimes suggest learning QiGong first. Not only are QiGong exercises easier to learn quickly, they also enhance the learning of T'ai Chi tremendously by building up your inner health before working on your outer health with T'ai Chi. QiGong also can help strengthen your ability to balance before you move into the slightly more complex T'ai Chi. The balancing subtleties in T'ai Chi are then more easily managed, which makes the flowing positions easier to learn.

QiGong likely had a large influence on the initial formation of T'ai Chi. Perhaps T'ai Chi, which was practiced in 500 B.C. was initially made up of QiGong but with more elaborate, larger movements and with more continuity: a dance to life, with liveliness coursing through the dancer. However it may have begun, T'ai Chi and QiGong have blended now to provide perfect companions for each other.

Many people ask whether QiGong can be done without any other exercise. Yes, it sure can. Probably the first QiGong practitioner thousands of years ago developed it just for the life-energy enhancement alone. This enhancement is certainly available through QiGong today. Some people who have limited movements find that QiGong is a full and complete exercise. Others go on to incorporate it into T'ai Chi. Keep in mind that the enhancement QiGong brings has made it a fundamental spiritual part of Buddhism, Taoism, Confucianism, and martial arts. Like T'ai Chi, it is a marvelous support for and a positive blend into anyone's life. Do it on its own or before, with, or after a run, walk, surf, or in conjunction with T'ai Chi.

ESSENTIALS

You can practice QiGong anywhere: in fresh air, under the blue sky, or greeting the day with the dew under your feet are the ancient ideals. If this works for you, great. If not, do it as you find best for you. You will need only clean air, space to move, and comfortable clothing.

You will likely be surprised at how easily you can learn QiGong. Not one position is difficult. The movements involve bending and straightening your legs, occasionally repositioning your legs, and making arm motions that are large and comfortable—all done with the breath.

Does QiGong Have Any Age Restrictions?

QiGong's appropriateness to any age is probably what I love best about it. Many types of exercise claim to be suitable for all ages, but it just isn't true (as seen in the number of running, yoga, climbing, biking, and even walking injuries).

- *Is your breath limited? Are you confined to a house, a chair, or a bed?* Do the movements as you can. Even for people unable to move below the neck, the breathing still has great value.
- *Are you sore, injured, or arthritic?* Let these activities join you as you are. Don't force.
- *Are you overly focused, unable to let down, buff but edgy, tense, or stressed?* Let the grace of movement teach you what true great health is.

QiGong (and T'ai Chi), when done easily and gently in harmony with your own abilities, will never harm you. These activities support your life as it is.

CHAPTER 2
The History of T'ai Chi and QiGong

The original words "T'ai Chi" come from the *I Ching* (*The Book of Changes*), in which the Chinese philosophy of Taoism was taught. Men spent their entire lives focusing on embodying spiritual truths, often choosing to live as hermits and monks.

Knowing Why the Practice Began

The very qualities that contributed to a more balanced life for a warrior also enhanced his fighting skills. Harmony, a calm attitude, and receptivity to increased mental clarity became aspects of martial arts to which warriors aspired. The warrior was able to blend this embodied art of inner harmony with the outer force of battle—to be in a warrior's conflict, conducting the business of war, but still filled with inner peace. They were in the midst of life while in the midst of death. It was into this need T'ai Chi Ch'uan (which is today's T'ai Chi coupled with martial arts) was born.

Understanding the Loss of Martial Arts from T'ai Chi Ch'uan

The healing art is known simply as T'ai Chi. Ch'uan, meaning "the fist," is dropped, leaving only "the supreme ultimate," the meaning of T'ai Chi. Masters of T'ai Chi Ch'uan generally believe that full benefits can't be derived from these sequential graceful movements without the Ch'uan component. They believe T'ai Chi will engender a general feeling of well-being, but the aspects of Ch'uan—speed, calmness, patience, courage, and perhaps even longevity will not be transmitted. For many, many people T'ai Chi offers fully satisfying benefits.

T'ai Chi has now evolved further into different forms. The Ch'uan has been left behind in some forms to focus on the T'ai Chi. I know of no other exercise that carries such a rich, flexible, and helpful tradition.

This book is about T'ai Chi, the healing aspects of T'ai Chi Ch'uan. For that reason we will be learning the Yang form. Should you at some time wish to investigate further the martial arts aspects of T'ai Chi Ch'uan, there is information in the back of the book to help you find schools and seminars on both T'ai Chi and T'ai Chi Ch'uan, as well as books, videos, and magazines.

FACTS

Masters of T'ai Chi Ch'uan generally believe that full benefits can't be derived from these sequential graceful movements without the Ch'uan (martial arts) component. They believe T'ai Chi will engender a general feeling of well-being, but the aspects of Ch'uan—speed, calmness, patience, courage, and perhaps even longevity will not be transmitted. For many people, however, T'ai Chi offers fully satisfying benefits, so the Ch'uan has been left behind in some forms to focus on the T'ai Chi.

Tracing T'ai Chi's Roots

The earliest references to T'ai Chi Ch'uan is when a Chinese hermit named Xu Xuan Ping practiced an art known as the Thirty-Seven Patterns of T'ai Chi Ch'uan. The first form was also called Changquan (Long Fist): named for the Yangtze River because the movement of T'ai Chi Ch'uan should be as long and continuous as the river. Very close to the same time, a Taoist priest from Wudang Mountain named Li Dao Zi practiced a similar physical movement. These first emergences of T'ai Chi occurred in the Tang Dynasty (A.D. 618 to 907).

The first time T'ai Chi Ch'uan was referenced in a classical text was in the writings of Chen Ling Xi in his manuscript, *The Method to Attain Enlightenment Through Observing the Scripture*. It was at this time T'ai Chi Ch'uan seems to have been blended into the monk-warrior traditions by men who were skillful in martial arts practice and spiritual development. It was then through the skills and observations of the priest Zhang San Feng that T'ai Chi Ch'uan came into full prominence.

Enter the Masters

Zhang San Feng (also spelled Chang San-feng) was a great master teacher who lived at the end of the Song Dynasty in the early twelve century. He was a graduate of the Shaolin Monastery, and then went on to continue his learning on Wudang Mountain in the Purple Summit Temple (just like in the movie *Crouching Tiger, Hidden Dragon*), a most revered temple of learning in the sacred mountains of Taoism. One day he had an opportunity to observe a fight between a snake and a bird (some say a crane; others, a sparrow). As the bird struck, the snake would avoid contact by using graceful, serpentine movements, waiting and swaying until it was ready to accurately strike. Watching this forceful but graceful combat, he was inspired to take what he had learned from observing the wisdom of nature and apply it to his own martial arts. He modified his harder, more outwardly forceful Shaolin Kungfu into a softer, more graceful style, the Wudang 32-Pattern Long Fist, which developed into T'ai Chi Ch'uan as we know it today.

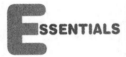

According to Chinese legend, human beings were given the great talent of being able to learn from every aspect of their environment. In this way, legend says, martial arts developed, from observation and imitation of the stillness of mountains, the fluidity of rivers, and the protective skills of the animals.

The Art Refines

Zhang San Feng was able to change the focus from martial arts (during training, warriors hit at sandbags, jabbed their palms into granules, and lifted many weights) and emphasize internal methods of control. T'ai Chi Ch'uan brought much subtlety to more classically combative movements. Included also was breath work (QiGong), chi channeling, and visualization. Zhang's movements then divided into three forms: Pakua Kungfu, Hsing Yi Kungfu, and T'ai Chi Ch'uan. (In this book we will be exploring only T'ai Chi Ch'uan, from which came T'ai Chi, which doesn't have a martial arts focus.)

The Lineage Develops

Zhang San Feng passed on his training to Taoist priest Taiyi Zhenren, who is still remembered as an accomplished Wudang swordsman. Taiyi, in turn, carefully imparted his knowledge. At the end of the Ming Dynasty, the Wudang Kungfu, which had been largely responsible for teaching T'ai

Chi Ch'uan to others, was no longer confined to teaching only the Taoist priests at the Purple Temple, but were now spreading the information through many secular disciples. Most historically interesting from the viewpoint of the T'ai Chi lineage was when Taoist priest and T'ai Chi Ch'uan master Ma Yun Cheng taught T'ai Chi Ch'uan to his favored disciple, Wang Zong Yue.

Wang Zong Yue in turn transmitted the art of T'ai Chi Ch'uan to another famous secular master, Zhang Sang Xi. It continued to pass through secular masters and disciples throughout China, but one theory holds it was probably Wang Zong Yue who taught the art to the powerful Chen family at their family settlement. The Chen family became great masters of T'ai Chi Ch'uan.

The Powerful Chen Family Enters

It was through the Chen family (who vary the history by claiming they learned it in the 1600s from their own ancestor, Chen Wang Ting) that the Chen style of T'ai Chi Ch'uan took form and spread. The contributions of this family rooted the destiny of T'ai Chi Ch'uan.

Yang Lu Chen (1799–1872) built the foundation of the Yang form of T'ai Chi Ch'uan. When a young man, he divested himself of all his possessions and went to work for the powerful Chen Chang Xin family in the Chen family compound to learn the secret art of T'ai Chi Ch'uan. He observed, in great personal secrecy, the transmitting of the form as it was taught by the patriarch master to family members and disciples. So adept was he at learning from watching that, unbeknownst to his employers, he attained a high standard with T'ai Chi Ch'uan.

Challengers would periodically appear at the Chen compound looking for a match. One particularly talented challenger beat not only the best disciple, but the most masterful Chen son. Seeking another challenge, he insisted on challenging the old man master of the Chen family. So determined was he that he called repeatedly on the compound with his demand. He was told that Sifu, the master, was on a prolonged trip. Undeterred, he refused to abandon his challenge. In China, honor was valued beyond anything else, so the family was at a loss as to how to save face because no one in the compound had a high enough standard of development to match him.

Feeling the desire to save the honor of the Chen clan, Yang Lu Chen stepped forward in peril of his life. Keep in mind that the entire Chinese upper class educational system was built on privacy, structure, and utmost secrecy. So seriously did they take this that violators who tried to be educated in their own right were killed. Yang Lu Chen stepped out of the servant rank and approached the challenger. He offered to share some Chen style T'ai Chi Ch'uan with him, stating his hope of being taught by the challenger. This was the honorable and polite way to ask for a challenge.

The Chens were, of course, shocked, even more so when the challenger was soundly defeated by Yang Lu Chen. While the Chens were likely glad that this adept challenger was defeated, their servant had violated laws that had to be enforced. Grave punishment was required. Everyone waited for Yang Lu Chen's appearance before the great Chen master/patriarch, Sifu Chen Chang Xin. All gathered in the family hall to watch Yang Lu Chen kneel before the master to apologize for stealing the secret arts and to await his punishment.

Sifu Chen Chang Xin offered Yan Lu Chen a cup of tea and sipped his tea in deep contemplation. "By accepting your tea and drinking it with me, I am accepting you as my disciple. In bringing honor to us, you've saved us from shame!" In that simple, compassionate act of inclusion, Sifu solved the problem.

Yang Lu Chen went on to further the Chen-style T'ai Chi Ch'uan, bring much honor to the Chen family, and spread the art of T'ai Chi Ch'uan.

The Three Forms of T'ai Chi Ch'uan

Within the Chen family, who maintained secrecy over their style of T'ai Chi Ch'uan, three styles, or forms, ultimately evolved. Each is unique, but still contains the overarching themes and foundations of T'ai Chi Ch'uan.

Old Form

The first is the Old Form. In this Old Form of T'ai Chi Ch'uan, the movement leads from the body to the arms. So for a punch, you would adjust your stance, letting the movement of your rotating body move into the arm. This creates and is characterized by large movements. The goal is to continually evolve into greater force.

New Form

In the New Form, the movement leads from arms to the body. The movement first comes from the arms. The body moves at the beckon of each arm according to the momentum of the punch. This form is faster in combat. For the body to follow the arm, a better flow of internal force is promoted.

Small Form

The third form, the Small Form, consists of a circular thrust of the punching arm. This creates a spiral force. This third form, which incorporates the force of the Old Form and the quicker movement of the New Form, is fast, conserves energy, and allows great balance to be maintained.

ESSENTIALS First learn the big form, then the new form, and finally the small form: Chen-style masters still believe that this is the best path of progression in learning both the strength and containment of martial art and the enhancement of health and inner harmony.

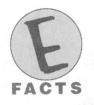

FACTS

In the mid-1800s, an old manuscript was found in a salt shop by a lucky scholar, who took it to his brother, Wu Yu Xiang, a student of T'ai Chi Ch'uan with the Chen clan. Wu, in turn, showed the manuscript to his friend and teacher, Yang Lu-shan. Yang, to his utter delight, confirmed the authenticity and wisdom of the manuscript. The manuscript is generally attributed to a great Wu Tang Mountain monk Zhang San Feng.

Choosing among the Four Branches of T'ai Chi

There are currently four different branches of the tree of T'ai Chi Ch'uan—each form has its own unique value:

- The Wu Style emphasizes small movement and body technique for combat.
- The Sun Style emphasizes high patterns and agile movements.
- The Chen Style emphasizes the hard and fast.
- The Yang Style emphasizes gentle, graceful movements for health.

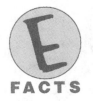

FACTS

The Yang School of T'ai Chi Ch'uan is named after the late Master Yang Cheng-Fu (1883–1936). His grandfather had taught it to his father then passed it on to the founder of the Yang school. Yang Cheng-Fu was greatly responsible for the dissemination of T'ai Chi throughout China, and overseas as well. After his death, his work was carried on by Tung Ying Chen and his eldest son, Yang Show-Chung.

Yang Lu Chen continued to be an advocate of equality in the transmittal of T'ai Chi Ch'uan. In his later years, he settled in Beijing and taught his Chen Style T'ai Chi Ch'uan far beyond the family members of the Chen family. Yang Lu Chen passed his knowledge on to his student

Wu Yu Xiang (18131–1880) and to his sons Yang Ban Hou (1837–1890) and Yang Jian Hou (1839–1917). His sons went on to evolve T'ai Chi Ch'uan into the Wu Style of T'ai Chi Ch'uan, which combines the Old Form and the New Form (see the preceding section). Wu Yu Xiang went on to develop the Sun Style T'ai Chi Ch'uan.

Yang Style is the commonly taught form in the Western world, and is, therefore, the form on which *The Everything*® *T'ai Chi and QiGong Book* focuses. Yang Style is probably the most popular form of T'ai Chi Ch'uan in the West today. The Yang Style enlarges and smoothes the movements that emphasize the graceful aspects of T'ai Chi Ch'uan. For this reason, it is sometimes called the Big Form. Yang Style has no foot stomping, punches, and so on. It is a pattern of slow, gentle grace, transforming T'ai Chi Ch'uan from a forceful martial art to the gentle health exercise of T'ai Chi.

How the West "Discovered" T'ai Chi

Many people remember the 1960s as a time of great changes in our country. One of the outcomes of this decade was a burgeoning interest in Eastern philosophies, healing methods, clothing, language, and so on. The upside of this proliferation of Eastern culture was that the influences of the East were strongly felt and disseminated. Of course, prior to this time, people had traveled in the East, loved it, and were affected by it, but it did not start its mainstream journey until the '60s. The downside of the quick proliferation of Eastern techniques throughout the West was a loss of quality in the transmission of the teaching due to enthusiastic—but often not well trained—instructors. One great strength in ancient China's teaching style was that it absolutely maintained the quality of T'ai Chi Ch'uan as it was being taught. One did not (would not!) consider teaching T'ai Chi Ch'uan unless a certain prescribed level of mastery had been attained, and that level of mastery was confirmed by esteemed masters. To take T'ai Chi Ch'uan lessons in China from a master who came from a long lineage of other T'ai Chi Ch'uan teachers was a different experience than learning T'ai Chi from a Westerner who had studied for a few years.

However, this proliferation of teachers, which would never have happened in ancient China's system, has extended the practice to the far reaches of the Western world. Another positive is that T'ai Chi without the Ch'uan evolved into being. The down side is that much of the precise disciplined aspects of the movements are often omitted. Western T'ai Chi is coming into its own, however, and we now have teachers who have studied the practice for decades, so the quality is improving. We are also lucky enough to have Chinese masters teaching through books, videos, seminars, and some personal sessions. China is a far more disciplined culture, and taking instruction from a T'ai Chi Ch'uan Chinese master is an important addition to any serious student's experience.

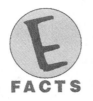
FACTS

When T'ai Chi was first practiced in the '60s, it was often seen as a hippie eccentricity. Its evolution throughout the last forty years shows T'ai Chi can still give great gifts, even if it isn't taught with classical perfection.

Letting the Masters Help You Today

Chinese masters were exclusive in both how they learned and how they taught T'ai Chi and QiGong. For centuries, the two practices were a part of the secret arts of Chinese warriors. They didn't want their enemies to know their trade secrets, and the whole experience of martial arts was dedicated to mastery over both self and an opponent. Having these secret disciplines of QiGong (internal force) and T'ai Chi Ch'uan (external strength) was a tremendous asset and not one to regard carelessly.

Two results evolved from this drive for privacy and excellence. The first was that methods were handed down very exclusively. One master chose a talented student and focused his knowledge and wisdom on him. The master might take in a few other disciples, but the group was kept exclusive. Second, because the teachings were so treasured, each master added his own wisdom to those who preceded him. This section focuses on some wise reflections on T'ai Chi from those ancient, wise martial artists.

Relaxation

There are several common themes in the guidance from the past. One is that relaxation is rewarded by T'ai Chi. This doesn't mean you must do a relaxation exercise before your class or practice. It simply means that as you do T'ai Chi, the overall focus is to relax into your body. You should feel a release down into your waist, or more accurately for our culture, your hip joints and pelvis. When the hip joints are loosened and the pelvis is relaxed, you can keep the lower body firm and stable and your feet grounded.

There is also an emphasis on having the body rebalanced so that the bottom is heavy and the top is light. In our culture, we tend toward the top being heavy and the bottom light. We also incline toward holding a great deal of tension in the hip joints and contracting the pelvis. This tension and contraction creates a situation where it becomes impossible for the chi to sink into the tan t'ien (see Chapter 1). Because the tan t'ien, also called the sea of energy, is the heart of T'ai Chi, these patterns are counter to the T'ai Chi and QiGong way. T'ai Chi and QiGong both emphasize relaxing into the body and dropping the breath and chi into the tan t'ien.

Improved Breathing

Just the improved breathing improves health. The breath becomes deeper and larger, which in turn brings more oxygen into the blood. The body also goes through a natural exercise when inhaling. Your chest expands and lifts, the lungs expand, the torso lengthens, the organs move a bit, the hips expand slightly, the spine lengthens, even the bony plates of your skull expand slightly. Our bodies were built to have this exercise several times a minute for our entire lives. We can all stop and take a deep breath when we think about it, but that may not be very often. QiGong and T'ai Chi teach you how to develop deep, relaxed breathing so effectively that your body is reminded to breathe deeply. If your body is fully reminded and indulged in this breathing, it will create a way to continue the experience.

Just as your body notifies you about thirst and hunger, it will do the same with breathing. After all, we can go much longer without either food or water than we can without air, so air is your first priority for being relaxed. It would be impossible to feel relaxed with a bare minimum of food or a few sips of water. This is the condition our bodies are in as a result of two things—faulty breathing habits and poor air quality.

ESSENTIALS

Who knows how much cultural stress we all carry just as a result of poor breathing. If you follow the masters' advice—sink into the tan t'ien by relaxing the pelvis and loosening your hip joints—you may find a whole new level of relaxation.

T'ai Chi and QiGong also emphasize the openness of the waist with movement. This is because the pelvis is the container for the tan t'ien. Not only can the chi not sink if the pelvis is contracted, but the container for the tan t'ien is not resilient. The hip joints provide the stability for the tan t'ien. It is through the hips, legs, and feet that the body stabilizes and grounds. If the pelvis is contracted and the hips are tight, the tan t'ien is denied chi, the container is non-resilient, and the tan t'ien is not stable. All of these create a condition of disease within the body. Loosening the hips, relaxing the pelvis, and dropping the chi into the tan t'ien gives your body what it needs to be healthier and more alive with energy/chi.

Balance

T'ai Chi and QiGong also emphasize that our bodies are a balance or a bridge between the earthly energies and the heavenly energies. The encouragement is to constantly be aware of this and always be assimilating vital energy from both heaven and earth. Heaven is the yang chi, earth is the yin chi, and tan t'ien is where they join if the chi is properly directed. This is energetic balance.

We also have physical or structural balance. You may think that standing balance—on your feet, gazing forward—would be the easiest thing in the world. It is actually not easy to simply stand in one place, unmoving, balanced between earth and heaven. This is usually a structural/muscular problem.

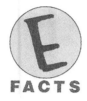

FACTS

Not only do we shorten our breath as we become adults, we also contort, to varying degrees, our body. Injuries, accidents, and prolonged stress all lay claim to throwing off the natural, easy balance we had as children. We don't arrive at unsteadiness in an instant. Poor balance develops over time as the injuries, accidents, and stress continue to hold the body in misalignment.

Healing from an injury or an accident doesn't in any way mean you've gotten your body back the way it was before. Those injured areas may be stiffer after they have completely healed. Stress builds upon itself, creating an unpleasant cycle of increasing stiffness and a slow, degenerating balance. T'ai Chi, one muscle at a time, one joint at a time, brings your body back to balance. T'ai Chi helps you reclaim your natural balance.

Quieting the Mind

Quieting the mind was the final emphasis of the ancients. Stilling the mind preceded contemplation, meditation, and T'ai Chi and QiGong. T'ai Chi is a movement meditation. Stillness of mind supports the benefits T'ai Chi makes available just as T'ai Chi promotes stillness of mind. Our minds are capable of thinking—having thoughts—and of mindfulness—experiencing no thoughts. T'ai Chi and QiGong seek to guide us on the path toward giving up in practice our thoughts and instead allowing the balance between earth and heaven we are bridging to lead us to mindfulness. Mindfulness is to be fully present in the experience of the moment with clarity and inner peace. Thoughts race into the past or the future. Mindfulness brings us into the present moment, relaxed and open, as if we were children.

Stillness

What each master wanted to achieve personally and pass on to a few treasured students was stillness in movement. By exercising, one creates a state of emotional stillness. A stillness that seems outside of regular time and separate from the busy day. It is this state of stillness that will benefit you with full spirit and rejuvenation. T'ai Chi can, in fact, like a sitting meditation, create a gate through which a world of stillness can be entered.

Spinal Health

The last area to be given special attention is the spine. The relaxed pelvis provides a container for the tan t'ien. Loosened hip joints and legs provide a stable, balanced ground. The spine is the super highway on which the chi runs. Connected to other energy centers in the body, the spine is where the chi courses to its destination. A flexible, agile, and free spine is essential for the resiliency of good health and well-being to enter your body, mind, and spirit. Ideally, you want your spine to move like a flexible cord, able to twist side to side, bend over easily, and roll up from a bent position with comfort.

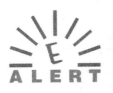

When loosening your spine, don't force; instead, give it time to find its flexible comfort. Imagine that you're breathing down the front of your spine when you inhale and that your breath is circulating up the back of your spine as you exhale. T'ai Chi allows you to loosen your spine as well as your hip joints.

CHAPTER 3

The Health Benefits of T'ai Chi and QiGong

T'ai Chi has always amazed people with the breadth and depth of its capacity to improve lives. Now, the health benefits of T'ai Chi are being studied by major medical research organizations: Johns Hopkins University has found that T'ai Chi lowers blood pressure; a National Institute on Aging study on falling accidents among the elderly found T'ai Chi to be the most effective prevention; other health studies have shown that it reduces stress.

The Physiological Effects

Both T'ai Chi and QiGong affect the human body in a variety of beneficial ways. You will improve your coordination, posture, breathing, skin tone, increase your mobility, decrease your blood pressure, tone your muscles, and even shed a few pounds. These physiological effects are discussed in the following sections.

Balanced Strength and Coordination

In the Western world, strength means a variety of things: Strength is often sought by bulking up the large muscles, usually through weight-lifting. Strength can also mean being strong in one's favorite sport. And strength often means getting strong in a few activities and having the heart strength to support them.

Eastern traditions focus on creating a great balance—strength and flexibility—throughout the body. Because in ancient China great battles were waged between districts, clans, and families (and even within families), the need for effective protection of the self was ever present. One had to fight with strength and suppleness to win. As the culture chose civilization over warring, these self-protection arts were improved into systems of martial arts. Then, as the martial arts became more and more refined, the disciplines became more intricate and sophisticated. One need only to look at an accomplished T'ai Chi practitioner or martial artist to see these principles in action. In the beginning, you may not leap 3 feet in the air and land silently like a cat, but you will find your walk and movements more graceful and your strength increasing.

Balanced strength and improved coordination occur because the positions incorporate all the muscles of the body appropriately, and the muscles strengthen in natural balance with one another. They give the support to one another as they were designed by nature to do. Their elasticity returns. Because you're working your body as it was meant to be worked—completely, thoroughly, and fluidly—the body relearns how to move without injury and remembers how to move with graceful, coordinated strength.

Improved Posture

When I was a child at a country fair in Ohio, a group of children were performing their ballet presentation on stage. I stopped to watch them for a minute and noticed their teacher, her back to me, on the side of the little stage. After the completion of the dance she turned with the dancers to receive the applause, and I was shocked to see she was an old woman. It fascinated me. Why did she look so young and vital from the back? I realized I had never seen anyone over sixty with great posture. And she certainly had it! She looked absolutely regal to me.

FACTS

Good posture allows our bodies to move properly. It also allows excellent blood circulation and great breathing. Over time, life can bow us. Work positions and life's challenges take a toll on how straight and confidently you stand.

T'ai Chi places great importance on the spine. The head is seen to balance delicately on the spine with light and free movements. The movements initiate at the tan t'ien so that the pelvis (or as the ancients spoke of it, the waist) is seen as supple and freely moving. The combination of these cornerstones of T'ai Chi movement create great posture. Your walk will become more erect, your step will be lighter. Your head will rest easily on your neck, and your pelvis or waist will move in an easy, graceful freedom. Good posture is a statement of mechanical efficiency. It is an eloquent statement of T'ai Chi's effectiveness!

Improved Breathing

Chi travels in electric currents that fill the air around you. We usually think of air as being empty, but in T'ai Chi, air is a full—even viscous—environment filled with a field of energy that connects us to the larger field of energy we call the universe. On these currents of chi is our life force. Without it, we die. When it diminishes from shallow breathing, we are less lively, and this usually registers as stress

The body relies totally on breath, oxygen, and chi for its well-being. The thought of being an effective martial artist or truly pursuing better health and well-being without good breathing is unthinkable. QiGong is all about breathing and creating new pathways to health through the breath. So you can safely assume that in your practice you will breathe more completely and perhaps resolve any breathing problems you may have.

In 1985, the Chinese government sponsored a research group (the Chi-Kung Scientific Research Society of China) to study the effects that QiGong creates in the body. It is through this type of effort that our Western desire to have data will be satisfied.

Increased Joint Flexibility

Dorothy, an eighty-year-old student new to T'ai Chi started the activity because of a femur broken just under the hip socket. This is a painful break and at eighty, a hard one to come back from. Her joints had become so stiff that she decided to try a modified version of T'ai Chi. Over a few months of diligent practice, not expecting the miracle of youth to suddenly descend upon her, she found that her joints were more flexible and her broken femur has healed nicely. Probably the best result is that her outlook became more positive because she was feeling less pain, experiencing less stiffness, and learning a new and valuable skill.

Increased Mobility

Jim, after having been a distance runner for many years, was finding that although running was a joy and a passion, it was not helping his overall mobility. His back was stiff, and although he stretched before each run, he still felt stiffness throughout his boy. His wife, May, had been taking T'ai Chi (he had teased that it was a pretty cushy exercise), and he decided to try it because he had seen such a change in her grace of movement. Sure enough, six weeks later, he was boasting of a flexibility and mobility that he had actually forgotten was possible. It had been so long since he had felt so smooth during and after his runs.

Toning of Muscles and Improved Weight Ratio

Bernie was your classic couch potato. He had a desk job, so his sharp brain was fully engaged, but his body sat in a chair, barely moving all day. He loved to eat, so dinner after work was a feast of pleasures to be followed by a quiet evening at home reading his favorite book before bed. Bernie didn't like to sweat, breathe heavily, or otherwise disturb his peaceful world. However, one day he took a good look at his girth in the mirror—it was sobering—and decided he would have to make a change. He loved his life and didn't want to stop anything. He hated exercise and thought it was menial and boring. But T'ai Chi struck him as peaceful and, perhaps, not boring, with no flowing sweat, so he tried it. The change over twelve months was dramatic. His skin was no longer pasty: It glowed. His paunch was gone. His breathing was no longer labored and heavy. He was still peaceful, loving his life and food and couch, but now he was healthy, too.

ESSENTIALS

The gentle rotating, opening, and shifting from side to side and back to forward can create a gentle, low-effort way to reduce pounds. Many students have found that T'ai Chi brings them a more normal (reduced) appetite as life energy is gained from the chi instead of relying heavily on food for that liveliness.

Improved Skin Tone

Because of the increase in circulation, the reduction in stress (which is responsible for early body aging), and plumping those meridians (chi highways throughout the body) up with yin/yang balanced chi, the skin glows when you regularly practice T'ai Chi. No matter what your skin color, the texture of the skin will likely improve. If you're light or light brown, your cheeks will get rosier. If you're black, your natural great skin texture will improve. Skin problems that occur in adolescents and prior to menstruation can sometimes be positively affected because of the rebalancing going on deep within the body. Organs function better, and this shows immediately in the skin. Deep breathing also is wonderful for your skin tone, texture, and color.

Lowered Blood Pressure

Hypertension (high blood pressure) can create deadly strokes. I have often heard over the years that practitioners have reduced their blood pressure or lowered the amount of medication they needed to control their condition. If you're going to start T'ai Chi in the hopes that you're one of the students who finds this true for you, do it wisely. Check with your doctor and take your blood pressure readings frequently.

Relief from Migraines

This claim is based on the experiences of T'ai Chi practitioners, not on scientific research. After a few months of practice, migraine sufferers may find a reduction in their painful symptoms. One reason may be the effects on circulation and quieting heightened nerve responses to life's challenges.

One remedy for migraine sufferers is to try to prevent the blood from engorging the brain and instead force it to be released into the arms and legs, which are often cold during an attack. T'ai Chi balances circulation.

E

FACTS

Migraines often occur in people who are quite sensitive by nature. All the sounds, pressures, sights, and speed of this world can be just a bit too stimulating to the nerves of sensitive people, who are often task-oriented, busy people who don't really take downtime. T'ai Chi provides a task that keeps the mind busy on something other than life's challenges and sounds, and over time, brings a deep balance to the whole system. Just letting this type of relaxation take hold at regular intervals allows the downward flow of chi to have more movement in the meridian system.

Whatever may happen to create the reduced symptoms is a blessing to anyone who has put up with the pain, nausea, and light sensitivity of migraines.

The Psychological Effects

Some of the psychological effects of T'ai Chi include relief from stress or depression, the ability to concentrate, a sense of spiritual awareness, and psychological help for fighting addiction. These benefits are discussed in the following sections.

Stress Prevention and Reduction

Tim is a counselor for adolescents, who need extra time and support to make it through those up and down years to adulthood. These kids are wonderful and demanding—high maintenance, so Tim can't possibly go to work, kick back, and give a halfhearted attempt. Each day he has to give 100 percent, and each day unexpected, often disturbing, experiences occur. Before he tried T'ai Chi, his stress level was mounting, and he was beginning to get sick with colds, flu, and so on.

In an attempt to find an outlet for some of the kids' excess energy and to encourage their interest in philosophy, he brought in a T'ai Chi teacher. This was a Western teacher who had adjusted aspects of T'ai Chi to the Western ideas of discipline. It suited some of the kids well. One student, who had been particularly hard to reach, seemed to be getting a lot from it. In an attempt to better bond with this child, Tim joined in the instruction. Tim found his stress melting. His attitude toward his job, its value, and his ability to make a difference became more clear to him. He started practicing twice a day. Both he and his student feel T'ai Chi has helped them a lot with stress. (See Chapter 15 for tips on getting kids to enjoy T'ai Chi practice.)

Increased Ability to Focus

The ability to focus is perhaps one of the greatest gifts being sought from T'ai Chi. The last decade has brought great technological change and with it, enormous amounts of information to understand. The computer age has changed the world as we have known it. This new world requires intense mental focus that has not been needed since the time of the great martial arts masters. Their need for discipline and mental mastery may have been in martial arts instead of technological arts, but the mental needs are similar. T'ai Chi focuses the mind and improves concentration just as well today as it did for Xu Xuan Ping, Zhang San Feng, and Taiyi Zhenren in the days of masterful, skillful martial arts (see Chapter 2).

Improved Spiritual Attunement

The word "spiritual" in the dictionary has several slightly different definitions. The definition that I want to work with here is one that relates to conscious thoughts, emotions, and spirit. T'ai Chi and QiGong attune or adjust the practitioner to his or her own conscious thoughts, emotions, and spirit.

T'ai Chi and QiGong support a personal faith, but aren't faiths in themselves. Even if you immerse yourself in the ideas of yin/yang, the five elements, and the I Ching, you're studying a philosophy, not a religion. The Tao itself is simply a sharing of ideas.

ESSENTIALS

> To do T'ai Chi and attune yourself spiritually means to decide to do a practice that by its very nature returns you more deeply to yourself and to all the layers of self that you have. Your centering into your body and mind through these activities attunes you to you. Your self-awareness increases in all four areas—body, mind, emotion, and spirit.

This is not to say you will become mired in self-absorption. To be self-absorbed is never to be able to be present with anything or anyone. The world becomes, in that case, a series of self-projections that serve only to process the introspection further. Instead, I mean self-awareness in the sense that you know how you feel in any given situation because you know your own feelings, and are so comfortable with them that you can feel what they tell you about yourself, but aren't ruled by your emotions. You appreciate them for their ability to connect you in empathy with the world around you. Your mind stays clear and unclouded by ruling emotions; your mind leads you through one life event after another.

You're calm, clear, unafraid, and yet deeply feeling—very human and connected.

You feel your soul/spirit as a daily part of your life. You probably know people who race through their lives like a chicken with its head cut off, so deeply involved with the details of life that they have no time for introspection, personal growth, and looking deeply and gratefully at what has been and is being learned. We also know wise people who seem to walk in a gracious, loving calm. Unflappable in stress, caring, concerned, and not pulled in a million different ways by life, they emanate a quiet courage and resiliency in their lives. Courage, resiliency, calm, wisdom, all these come from one source: self-awareness, the knowledge of one's own nature.

Self-awareness brings the ability to take full responsibility for one's actions and view then with understanding. It fits people anywhere, anytime, in any faith. As T'ai Chi practice deepens the awareness of one's self, and the body and mind unite in clarity, the spirit within is also made clear. (See Chapter 19 for more on spirituality.)

Depression Relief

Certain types of depression respond to T'ai Chi and QiGong. If you're on medication, however, make a joint decision with your doctor about T'ai Chi's value and how best to avail yourself of its potential for you.

There are increasing statements from students that the feeling of calm and oneness that emerges from T'ai Chi postures and movements bring a greater feeling of balance and a relief from the loneliness of depression.

Decline of Substance Abuse

I have no experience with this particular benefit, and although anecdotal evidence exists, research does not. However, many people with substance abuse problems begin the abusive cycle because of depression or mood disorders. If T'ai Chi and QiGong can reach in and balance these to some degree, people may feel less of a need to rely on substances.

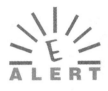

ALERT

The return of health and balance to the body/mind will create a diminished desire to fulfill cravings, perhaps even substance abuses. As the body becomes healthier, the physical cravings may become more manageable. With counseling and support, T'ai Chi students have learned healthier and happier ways to enliven and excite their lives.

Emptying Your Cup

An oft-told story tells of an educated man coming before a master teacher. "Hello," he said, "my name is Professor Smith. I am a graduate of three universities and have authored books, articles, and research papers. I would very much like to learn from you."

"Won't you sit down?" invited the master.

"Thank you," the educated man replied as he sat upon a pillow near the teacher.

"Would you like some tea?" the master asked of him.

"Thank you, I would," the professor replied.

The master started pouring the tea into the professor's cup and continued pouring the tea until it spilled over the edges of his cup and into the saucer. Filling the saucer, he continued to pour as it spilled onto the table. Finally the astonished professor could hold back no longer. "My cup is full and the tea is spilling everywhere!"

The master looked at him, paused in his pouring, and said, "Yes, you come with a full cup. Your cup is already spilling over, so how can I give you anything? Come with emptiness, openness, or I can give you nothing."

Before a T'ai Chi or QiGong class or a practice, empty your cup. Let the day release. Let what you're holding onto drop away. Feel yourself begin to empty, to open and receive. Give up your preconceptions about what your practice time is going to bring you.

In Western culture, the body is usually doing one thing and the mind is doing another. Enormous amounts of stress build up as a result of these two different experiences going on at the same time. We have virtually no exercise or mental effort that unites the two in a single, unified action, and yet the best way to reduce stress is to combine mind and body. Ten minutes of doing something where the body/mind are working together is more relaxing than two hours of activities that keep them separate.

FACTS

Good body/mind activities include cooking, gardening, model car building, and so on. Each offers an opportunity to unify the thought and the action. Will the mind drift? Sure. But the action you're involved in—cooking, gardening, model car building— will call the mind back as incidents that require attention.

T'ai Chi and QiGong also join body and mind. As you learn and become more comfortable with the movement in practice, you will feel the same relaxation that occurs when your body and mind are absorbed. But with T'ai Chi and QiGong, you have the enormous added value of being involved in an ancient discipline that doesn't just stop with body/mind harmony. T'ai Chi and QiGong fuel the chi, balance the yin and yang, and produce an array of health benefits that exceed any other single activity. The irony is that for an activity so full of gifts, as the master teacher says, you must come to it empty in order to know the fullness. Practice emptying your cup. As best as you can, do the following:

- Empty thoughts
- Empty expectations
- Empty performance

- Empty anxiety
- Empty comparison
- Empty competition

Becoming Resilient

Resilience is a wonderful word. It means the ability to return to an original form after being bent, compressed, or stretched; the ability to recover from an illness, depression, adversity, or the like; and the ability to spring back or rebound.

When you've had a bad day, a life challenge, or just a busy life, the stress of it shows in the tense muscles in your shoulders, legs, wrists, back, ankles, and so on. It would be great if we could regain this natural elasticity with deep sleep alone, but this is not enough. As children, we rebalance in sleep for twelve to thirteen hours. As adults, however, the latest studies show that many people now get six or fewer hours of sleep.

This lack of sleep is from our lives being so full. By the time you do everything you're committed to, it is late at night, and to continue the commitments, you have to arise at an early time. This says nothing of interrupted sleep from cheap car alarms, sick babies, anxious thoughts, indigestion, poor health, low estrogen—the list is endless! In the precious few hours that remain, you just don't have enough time for your body to completely unwind, for your unconscious to work out the day through dreams, for you to seek and find the rebalancing of body, mind, and spirit that deep sleep brings.

With the diminishment of deep and restful sleep comes a diminishment of resilience. The days hit you harder. You get less pleasure from your activities. You run, work out, do yoga, but that deep lack of resilience continues to build. This need for resilience may be one of the most valuable assets of T'ai Chi and QiGong. T'ai Chi puts the emphasis on softness and flexibility, lightness and agility in movement. As resilience returns to the body, you don't depend so completely on sleep to take care of all your stress; instead, you have helped by doing twenty minutes of T'ai Chi. You have found another route to rebalance and rebound. As a result, you will awaken from limited or disturbed sleep more refreshed, having found resiliency in both sleep and in T'ai Chi.

Slowing Down

Your life is full. People rush from place to place and commitment to commitment, wishing for simplicity and a less hurried life. I live in a town that was for many years a sanctuary of peace and simplicity. In the past few years a large influx of people who want the peace and simplicity have moved in. Our newcomers, however, aren't equipped with the behavior to adjust themselves to our peace and simplicity. They lack the behaviors necessary to learn from the community about how to live more peacefully, more simply, and more meaningfully. As a result, drivers are now much more rude and demanding, and the town is losing its closeness in the me-first, you're-in-my-way attitude of our new town members. They don't know how to nourish the fountain they draw from and, as a result, the fountain is diminishing.

Everyone probably longs to have a life that is richer and happier, with meaningful work, well adjusted kids, long-term friends, and a loving family and/or partner. These are needs that run across all humanity. But our built-up stress, our inability to rebound into a fresh and open emptiness each day, and the complexity of our lives have become enormous problems that stand in our way. Or perhaps we could also say that we stand in our way.

In order to achieve the level of contentment you want, you need effective tools for becoming truly resilient. QiGong and T'ai Chi assist in this effort in the most helpful of ways. The lightness of the moves restores resiliency to joints and muscles, the breath cultivates and nourishes the chi, the disciplined style of motion balances the yin/yang within. Sleep becomes enough. T'ai Chi and QiGong become assets to rebounding from the myriad events of a day. Your sense of well-being strengthens. Your feeling of harmony and balance in the world is more apparent. Your patience with others is easy. No one is in your way. Your life is not unmanageable. Your stress has melted into rest. The life fountain of pleasure, joyful simplicity, and rich meaning is yours to draw from because you're refilling it each day. Only an ancient form of movement could give so much.

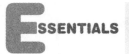

It makes no matter whether you are a martial arts master or a schoolteacher, the goal for a rewarding life is the same. The reason these exercises have endured for thousands of years is because they deliver. They delivered then, and they deliver now. If anything, after having been honed by time, they deliver better now than ever before.

CHAPTER 4

The Philosophical Aspects of T'ai Chi and QiGong

The philosophical aspects of T'ai Chi can be difficult to express in a linear language—but this chapter gives it a try! The value and therapeutic potential of T'ai Chi, along with the tremendous growth it is now experiencing worldwide, are examples of the riches the practice carries for us. T'ai Chi, the movement, is the messenger of the philosophy of the Tao.

T'ai Chi Is a Movement Philosophy

T'ai Chi is not a religion. It is a movement that has been evolving over centuries. T'ai Chi movement engages the practitioner's body, mind, and spirit in a great wholeness, oneness, or nothingness (called Wu Chi) as it divides at T'ai Chi—the energy moment—into yin and yang energy flows. It is for this reason that T'ai Chi and QiGong support any faith or belief system. A good analogy may be that if you take a deep breath of fresh air and have a good stretch, anything you decide to do is enhanced. T'ai Chi and QiGong have been used in China, however, to understand better the faith of Taoism.

The Wu Chi, or the Source of All

Taoism is an encompassing faith that embraces the concept of the completeness and wholeness that is at the same time the unknowable nothingness called Wu Chi. Everything in the universe is believed to evolve continually from this unknowable but accessible source. The purpose of life is to live in embodied balance, drawing from the source of wholeness, oneness, or nothingness. All actions of life are prisms through which we can experience the Tao's wholeness— health, medicine, communication, meditation, arts and music, business, and so on.

ESSENTIALS

Anything you can think of is a part of the Tao. Each movement of or into life is realized as a great potential for a personal experience of oneness. Each moment of life is permeated with a gift that embodies a deep sense of being connected to the Wu Chi, and that sense of connectedness can be embodied by anyone.

Balance is the key. The personal experience of health and well-being become ways to finding the wholeness—or the nothingness—or letting it find you. At the same time, this balance can be expressed through the practitioner in the moment of T'ai Chi. To become able to engage this source, Wu Chi, as a continual awareness in one's daily life, was the expression of a life lived in perfection. The perfect, nimble expression of balance was the illumination of the soul shining through the personality.

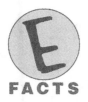

FACTS

Every human behavior is a lens through which the Wu Chi flows into yin and yang (through T'ai Chi). T'ai Chi in this sense isn't restricted to just the positions you're learning in this book. T'ai Chi in this sense means that moment when stillness becomes movement. In this way the moving leaf, trotting horse, a quick smile, and gentle wind are all T'ai Chi.

The Wholeness Divides

T'ai Chi is where the Wu Chi divides into yin and yang. Everything in nature becomes a part of and is intertwined by these two forces of energy. Everything is included by Yin, the feminine, and yang, the masculine, and they are included in everything. Yin and yang represent and express the natural harmonious polarity of all life.

Everything in matter is subject to incline (or growth) and decline (or decay). All things, even the smallest, are growing one step at a time in an astonishing process of order and constant change. Your body, being an important part of nature, involves and expresses the properties of yin and yang. These are complementary polarities that divide at T'ai Chi and then direct themselves into unifying in all forms of life. All phenomena, including everything that happens within your body, involve the interaction of these two energy forces.

Chi is spirited vitality (or energy) from the universe—wholeness or nothingness, the force within which the yin and yang flow. Your health and well-being depend upon how these flows move through your body. Yang flow is warm and active. Yin force is cool and receptive. You are affected by the amount of chi you've cultivated within and how the chi is circulating through the energy meridians of the body. The chi is cultivated and stored in the pelvic tan t'ien (see Chapter 1).

T'ai Chi also moves to create an inner environment for the proper balance of yin and yang. These flows are within the chi and move throughout the whole body, instilling the correct balance of yin and yang energy force in each organ of the body as well as the meridian system. This meridian system circulates like little highways within the entire body. When the life force of chi is obstructed or when the balance of yin and yang within the organ is upset, illness occurs.

ESSENTIALS

T'ai Chi and QiGong support the cultivation of chi and continuing proper balance of yin-yang throughout the body. By doing both activities on a regular basis, unwanted obstruction of the meridians (chi highways throughout the body) and yin-yang imbalances in the organs is avoided or corrected.

Wu Chi is the wholeness or the nothingness, and T'ai Chi is the moment when movement allows the division of yin and yang to occur. This describes not only the aspects of universal creation, but also initial stages of all relationships. For example, prior to a person entering an empty room, it is the Wu Chi. As soon as the person enters and brings movement, T'ai Chi begins. T'ai Chi is then the source point for yin and yang to emerge. A harp with no player is Wu Chi. When the musician plays, it is T'ai Chi; the movement has begun, and yin and yang express the complementary polarities that, when balanced, unite to form a whole. Wu Chi then exists before anything happens. The intention to create movement arises from Wu Chi. When something arises from Wu Chi and the original state of nothingness is altered, T'ai Chi begins.

FIGURE 4-1

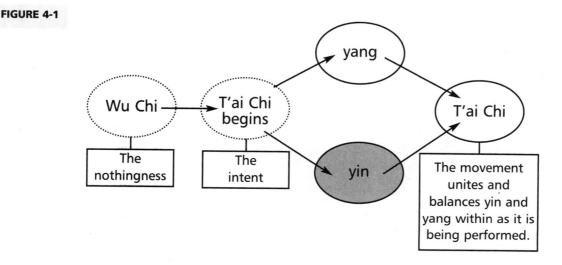

FIGURE 4-1 diagrams the Wu Chi, the beginning of T'ai Chi, yin and yang, and the movement T'ai Chi. This figure is an attempt to illustrate the energy force of the great emptiness/or the great potential as it is activated through intent at the beginning of T'ai Chi. The intent divides into yin and yang, according to the nature of the intent. Yin/yang, the balanced opposites, unite in T'ai Chi.

ALERT

When yin-yang emerge to unite in T'ai Chi, the level of balance or equality that occurs has to do with the nature of the intent that created the emerging flow. An angry mood or intent will carry more yang. A sad mood will carry more yin into the uniting. T'ai Chi is about restoring balance or equality within your daily life so you do not have excess yang or yin.

By bringing your mind, body, and spirit into the place where these energies unite, in harmony with the flows of yang and yin, you teach your mind, body, and spirit how to engage these flows in an equal unity. Your T'ai Chi movement embodies the T'ai Chi. This balance that occurs as a result of joining the flows with your own T'ai Chi will then affect your moods, thoughts, spiritual development, and body health. This potential for balanced interaction of force and receptivity is within your body, and will then be within your life.

FIGURE 4-2

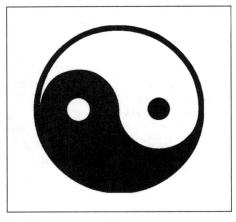

T'ai Chi is a movement meditation that balances and equalizes yin and yang as the uniting is happening within the body. This uniting within the body goes on ceaselessly. In fact, the Chinese belief is that the yin and the yang are always joining within you. You can't cease this uniting and also be alive, because the chi yin/yang is the very essence of life. It and you create your animation and liveliness according to your personal yin-yang balance, which, of course, changes constantly. This balance of yin and yang is shown in **FIGURE 4-2**: Within yang is the seed of yin; within yin is the seed of yang.

Suppose you lift weights, and you have bulk in your muscles. You're strong in these muscles, on the outside layers of your body, but you have had no inner training to match the emphasis on outer strength. You have had no instruction on how to develop your internal force. (This is the central theme in all martial arts—to cultivate, master, and direct your chi, which is your internal force.) You need more yin, so your yin and yang balance, then, would look like **FIGURE 4-3**.

FIGURE 4-3
FIGURE 4-4

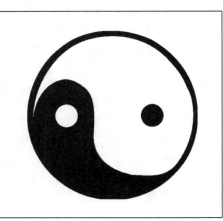
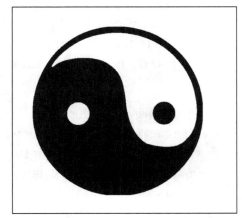

Now suppose you are timid. As a result, you have developed a lifestyle that is retreating. You develop your inner world but are only truly comfortable in the privacy of your own home. You would be uniting yin and yang within you with an overabundance of yin. You need more yang—see **FIGURE 4-4**.

ESSENTIALS

The Chinese believe that keeping the yin and yang in balance is the essence of youth, health, and well-being. The entire eternal cycle of life is designed to understand the two flows of essential chi and watch and record their tremendous influence.

So both a well-muscled (but poorly inner-developed) and inner-developed (but timid) person decide to take T'ai Chi. The well-muscled person with too much yang learns about internal force—the quiet, receptive center within that's filled with personal stillness. The power of receptivity shows more clearly when to step in and act and when to step back and allow. A new sense of confidence enters. There will be, perhaps, less conflict, less need to maintain power over others, and an easier, more relaxed time with other people. The self-consciousness, as opposed to self-awareness, will diminish and with it, any inappropriate competitive, defensive, or demanding inclinations. This will all occur with no diminishment of power. Actually, the act of power, focus, and protection will become more effective. The yin-yang balance will look again like **FIGURE 4-2**.

For the timid person with too much yin, the desire or need to retreat to feel confident and comfortable with oneself and life will begin to change. As yin and yang unite under the direction of the T'ai Chi, new awareness will occur. A new inner confidence, one that emanates outwardly (yang) will grow and create a realization of inner confidence but not just at home. It radiates outward, drawing a forward movement into life in a new way. Life seems more engaging, interesting, not simply "too intense." Life is expanding, and more comfort and confidence is occurring. Released outer force has brought a needed and welcomed balance. The yin and yang now looks more like **FIGURE 4-2**.

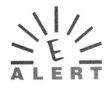

Balanced yin and yang energies are vital for good health—people become sick when this balance is broken. The circular movements of T'ai Chi mirror this important balance. These physical activities also necessarily involve internal work, because mind and body participate in the same energies.

The Five Elements Interact

Yin and yang and the balance you achieve with them has great effect on all parts of you. Emotional, physical, mental, and spiritual health are all guided by them. In keeping with this concept, Chinese medicine observes five elements: water, fire, wood, metal, and earth. The elements, because they spring from nature, may seem separate from us, but they are considered to be a dynamic process that was basic in understanding the movements of and through nature, people included. These elements are seen as dynamic, interactive, and that from which all life is made. Each element carries its own unique qualities:

- **Water:** Soaks and descends.
- **Fire:** Heats and moves upward.
- **Wood:** Can be formed.
- **Metal:** Melting, molded, and hardened.
- **Earth:** Provides nourishment through sowing and reaping.

As these five elements interact and are changed by the interaction, four major principles come forth: mutual creation, mutual closeness, mutual destruction, mutual fire. The dynamic interactions are discussed in the following sections.

Mutual Creation

One element produces the other in an endless cycle of creation.

- **Wood creates fire:** By rubbing two sticks together, fire occurs.
- **Fire creates earth:** As fire burns, ash is created and the ash becomes earth.

- **Earth creates metal:** Metal is found within the earth.
- **Metal creates water:** Dew forms on metal left out at night (this dew water was often used in healing) and at high temperatures, metal melts into liquid.
- **Water creates wood:** Water nourishes the trees that become wood.

This is a cycle of creation—see **FIGURE 4-5**. You can enter the cycle at any point.

FIGURE 4-5

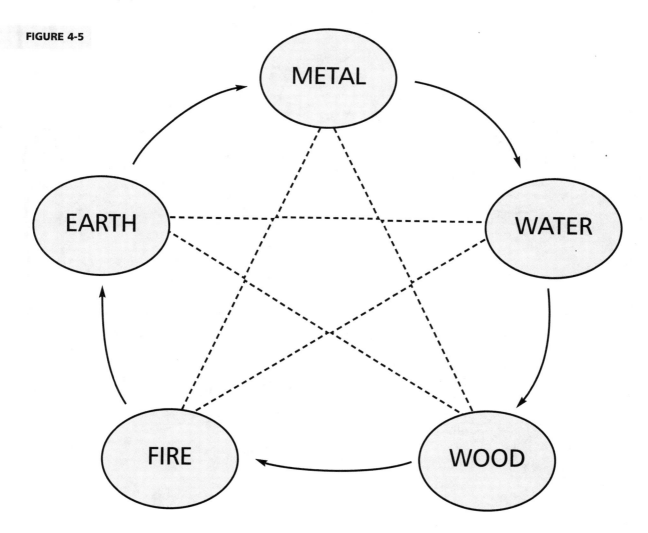

Mutual Closeness

Wood is close to water. Water is close to metal. Metal is close to earth. Earth is close to fire. Fire is close to wood. This relationship is not unlike a mother and child: a natural, organic closeness of the element to its creator.

FIGURE 4-6

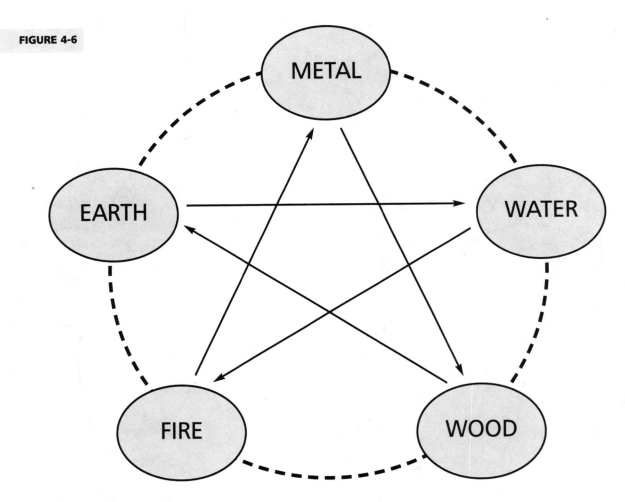

Mutual Destruction

This principle presents the conflicts that erupt between elements (see **FIGURE 4-6**):

- **Wood weakens earth:** Wood leaches elements from earth.
- **Earth limits water:** Earth contains water's movement, as in lakes and dams.
- **Water extinguishes fire.**
- **Fire conquers metal:** Fire weakens metal's great strength by melting it.
- **Metal destroys wood by chopping it down.**

Mutual Fear

Based on the mutual destruction in the preceding section, each element has a respect for or a fear of the element that has the ability to destroy it: Earth fears wood, because wood weakens earth nourishment. Water fears earth, because earth contains water. Fire fears water, because water extinguishes fire. Metal fears fire, because fire melts metal. Wood fears metal, because metal cuts wood.

People Share Traits with the Five Elements

People are also seen to be made up of the five elements. The composition or interaction of these elements make up the nature of the person, give clues to self-understanding and knowing other people better, and give vital information about the best route to health.

The elements and how they affect us is complex, but a very simple summary is as follows:

- **Wood:** An active, direct person
- **Metal:** A contained person
- **Fire:** An intense, quick-to-respond person
- **Water:** An emotional person
- **Earth:** A solid, nurturing person

As in all of the wholeness of the Tao, these principles govern or provide guidelines for the Chinese approach to healing or medicine. These principles of the five elements and the guidelines that come from the principles are applied to physiology, pathology, diagnosis, and therapy.

In diagnosing or understanding imbalances that are then believed to contribute to disease, the organs of the body are divided into: yin—solid organs; yang—hollow organs. Each organ has an element:

- **Heart:** Fire
- **Spleen:** Earth
- **Lungs:** Metal
- **Kidney:** Water
- **Liver:** Wood

- **Small intestine:** Fire
- **Stomach:** Earth
- **Large intestine:** Metal
- **Bladder:** Water
- **Gall Bladder:** Wood

This theory of the five elements and their relationship to one another throughout all of life—people and events—has been used in Chinese medicine to maintain health and cure illness. So deeply did these ancient doctors believe in the value of their abilities to create health using this model that they are said to have accepted payment only when able to keep the patient well. If the patient became diseased, the doctor took no payment until health or balance had returned. If this lore is true, it points out the mutual partnership of the doctor/patient relationship. The patient was regular, committed, and conscientious in following the guidelines of health and balance the doctor laid out. The doctor accepted full responsibility if the outlined program worked. This type of equal and mutual partnership in the maintenance of health is wonderful to consider.

ESSENTIALS

T'ai Chi and QiGong, of course, are fundamental in this approach to being in harmony and health in the eternal cycle of life. Your capacity is directly related to the amount of chi you have circulating within.

The five elements provide a structure for understanding how the aspects of nature, seasons, colors, and flavors correspond to organs of your body.

TABLE 4-1

THE FIVE ELEMENTS AND ASPECTS OF NATURE

	WOOD	FIRE	EARTH	METAL	WATER
Direction	East	South	Center	West	North
Season	Spring	Summer	Long summer	Fall	Winter
Color	Blue	Red	Yellow	White	Black
Flavor	Sour	Bitter	Sweet	Acidic	Salty
Organ	Liver	Heart	Spleen	Lung	Kidney
Sensory organ	Eye	Tongue	Mouth	Nose	Ear

You can see in **TABLE 4-1** what each element governs and how the interrelationships are defined. Seeing this as an interrelationship rather than singular functioning (which is usual in Western medicine, where, for example, we treat one organ for an illness), the Chinese doctors treat the whole body.

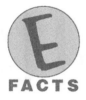

FACTS

The concepts of mutual creation and mutual destruction are applied in a very intricate, sophisticated theory that takes years to learn properly. This theory explains how low functioning or deficiency in one organ can (and usually does) create a malfunctioning of another organ or in several organs.

The belief is that bringing balance to the dysfunctional organ restores balance in the entire body. This intricate system of rebalancing is usually not achieved simply by taking some medicine. Instead, the solution approaches the imbalance from a whole perspective. The five elements and how they apply to everything is understood through the various relationships that can exist—creative, close, destructive, fearful.

Once the five-element interaction source of the health problem is uncovered, various tools are applied to create a balance. Acupuncture and acupressure points are stimulated along the meridians (chi highways throughout the body) to level chi flow. Herbal remedies are given to bolster the body's reserves and give nourishment where needed.

Breathing instructions are given through QiGong. T'ai Chi is recommended for exercise. Attitude adjustments are suggested, too.

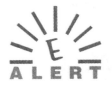

ALERT

Arts, music, silence, and meditation are all part of a program of lifelong health. Everything in life that you are affected by is analyzed from the perspective of your attitude toward the event and whether your attitude balances or unbalances you.

Spreading Positive Energy Through T'ai Chi

Any person who has traveled to the East, particularly China, has noticed groups of people doing T'ai Chi together. Sometimes large groups of people are doing QiGong and T'ai Chi together. (Now that T'ai Chi is so well known throughout the world, this is being seen more and more everywhere.) These are people of all ages. T'ai Chi is done in every local park, morning and evening. The Chinese consider themselves to be a very positive people, effective at achieving their goals, and T'ai Chi is seen as an activity essential to this positive attitude.

As the chi is gathered and cultivated in the tan t'ien (see Chapter 1), it is then dispersed throughout the body. The chi now differentiates into yin and yang flows through meridians. Twelve meridians run throughout the body like energy highways. Each meridian is associated with an organ. The name of the organ (lung, liver, and so on) refers to the physical organ and to the whole system of energy. Each organ has a unique energy flow, and it is this flow that runs in the meridians.

The meridians pass through the entire body: head, trunk, arms, and legs. All along these energy highways of specialized yin and yang are points that respond to stimulation. These are precise locations that are used to regulate the energy flow and, therefore, the functioning of the organ/meridian system. These meridians are regulated through acupuncture and acupressure, but even more so through QiGong and T'ai Chi practices.

T'ai Chi was developed to precisely harmonize these flows as the T'ai Chi positions are accomplished. Each step and hand movement is designed to put the meridian flows into accord with one another and with the larger universal system of energy flows. Each position has been given an element/meridian:

- **A forward step:** Metal
- **A withdraw step:** Wood
- **Looking left:** Water
- **Looking right:** Fire
- **Central equilibrium:** Earth

ESSENTIALS

The T'ai Chi movements are precisely designed to promote the correct energetic balance of the internal organs. It is no wonder so many people practice T'ai Chi daily or why so many new learners are jumping on board each day!

T'ai Chi and the *I Ching*

The words "T'ai Chi" come originally from the *I Ching*. The motion of life is the T'ai Chi of life, and yin and yang flow through each aspect of life, bodies, nature, and events. When you embody an understanding of this yin and yang flowing through all things, you can begin to understand how to view everything from the wisdom of this perspective of change/balance/change/balance.

The *I Ching* has been called many things—an oracle, a guide, and a reflection of one's unconscious are a few. It is a wonderful book that imparts reflections on the action and interaction of yin and yang in the seeker's life. The *I Ching*, then, is a guidebook and is available at any bookstore.

For more centuries than we can identify, the *I Ching* has been in China utilized as a tool for wiser living. It was distinctly Chinese until the 1800s when a Christian missionary named Richard Wilhelm traveled to China. He was a deeply religious man and very interested in the religion he taught, but also in the people he was teaching. He taught them about Jesus' love and over time, his Chinese friends taught him about Taoism. They also showed him the *I Ching*. They studied his way, and he became interested in theirs. Over time, he was so taken by the philosophic and metaphoric guidance of the *I Ching* that he took it upon himself to translate it from Chinese to English. Chinese, however, isn't easily molded into English. This was a huge task, a great responsibility, and became a great gift to the mutual understandings of two great faiths.

Upon returning to his native Germany, Wilhelm introduced the *I Ching* to German physician and forefather of psychology, Carl Jung (pronounced "yung"). Jung was immediately also taken by this wise and mysterious book. He was particularly interested in its understanding of synchronicity within the fabric of life events. Jung further engaged and extended the potential importance of the book by writing an interesting introduction to it.

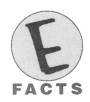

FACTS

The *I Ching* continues to stand as a work of great philosophical value worldwide. Its pertinence to T'ai Chi and QiGong is that it is a deeper look at the forces of yin and yang in life events. To cultivate chi, balance yin and yang, and grace your life with the movements of T'ai Chi, a wise and ancient look at the power of these forces in all of life makes sense.

CHAPTER 5

T'ai Chi and Your Chi/Breath

The ancient Chinese believed, and many people today agree, that the life-giving and life-sustaining force is within our breath, and that when we breathe, we take in this force (also called the engine of life) into our bodies. The air goes into the lungs, the oxygen circulates through the blood, and chi circulates throughout the body on energy highways.

Understanding the Need for Breathing Exercises

Just as breath is stored in the lungs, chi is stored in the tan t'ien, a place deep in the pelvis that's one and one-third inches below the navel in the center of the pelvis. All breath work is designed to fill, store, and finally cultivate chi in the tan t'ien. For this reason, all the breath exercises carry as their single purpose the goal of gaining control over your chi.

The Chinese name for this was Tao-Yie. This is the name given by the ancient Taoists to the concept of developing energetically the outside and the inside of the body. Tao means outside development, having to do with the T'ai Chi, or movement. Because T'ai Chi moves every joint, it promotes optimum circulation of blood and oxygen throughout the body. Yie means inside development, and this is entirely involved with the promotion of chi so every part of the body is infused with life-giving, health-promoting chi. T'ai Chi has had both of these benefits intertwined from ancient times.

The Practice of To Noa

The Chinese word for breathing exercises—not QiGong, which is an entire skill in its own right—is To Noa. "To" means to exhale carbon dioxide. "Noa" is to inhale fresh air. To Noa, then, implies two areas of value that are being taught. The first is the practice itself, the actual bare-bones instruction. The second, and perhaps the more intriguing, is the set of methods that actually let the breath and chi penetrate every part of the entire body.

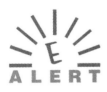
ALERT

Breathing is only half the plan. In order to have optimum health and well-being, you must be also creating an inner environment where the chi can penetrate even the most resistant spot. These areas that would not ordinarily have an abundance of chi are the areas that become most vulnerable to injury and disease.

Breathing Properly

In Chapter 12, you're introduced to QiGong breathing skills. In this section, I give you just the tip of the iceberg about breathing skills.

T'ai Chi is based on your most natural breathing. Slow, gentle, and deep, it increases lung capacity and expands the organs, so that oxygen fills the body on the inhale. When you exhale, carbon dioxide exits, freeing the body's cells of waste products.

Unless otherwise instructed, breathe in through your nose, but call your breath into the body through the tan t'ien, not the nose, then to the perineum, up the spine, and out the nose on the exhale while the chi flows down the front in the tan t'ien. If the tan t'ien is not involved, which means you expand the lower lungs and abdomen out on the inhale and in on the exhale, your breath is shallow in the lungs and your chest is tense. Your body then loses its natural center of gravity. This is one of the most common reasons for tension and the fatigue that results.

ESSENTIALS
To get your body back in balance during a stressful day, take a minute and do some T'ai Chi/QiGong breathing. A few moments will settle you down. Because of your body muscle memory, the more frequently you interject T'ai Chi and QiGong breath into your day, the more quickly and effectively you will feel the effects.

Many people find that when they start T'ai Chi and QiGong, their need for sleep diminishes naturally: They either stay up longer or get up earlier. Either way, people practicing T'ai Chi and QiGong feel refreshed after sleep, and this feeling of being well-rested lasts throughout the day. The reason for this is simple: Because of the natural orientation of T'ai Chi and QiGong, the body has the oxygen and chi it needs to run smoothly and effectively.

If your car is running poorly and provides unreliable transportation throughout your day, it is a constant stressor. You're less able to be fully present in the opportunities the day is offering because of your poorly running car. But when your car is running perfectly, what a pleasure it is to be moved from place to place so easily. How wonderfully it opens up life and options to you. So it is with your body.

Prebirth Breath

A breathing style I consider especially valuable is the prebirth breath. When used during the day along with just plain-old regular breathing, a nice development of breath and chi occurs. This practice was used as part of ancient T'ai Chi training, and you can use it as your teacher instructs and also as a part of your everyday life.

Reverse Breathing

This form of breathing is also called reverse breathing, because the abdomen contracts on the inhale and expands on the exhalation. (In normal breathing, the reverse occurs.)

The value the ancient T'ai Chi students placed on the prebirth or reverse breathing was great. Their theory is that prebirth breathing imitates the natural breath when one is in his or her mother's womb. Nourishment and oxygen come through the umbilical cord, and carbon dioxide and toxins are eliminated through it. The fetus must draw in the lower abdomen in order to draw in oxygen and must push out carbon dioxide and waste products. When the umbilical cord is severed at birth, "normal" breathing begins.

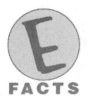

FACTS

The prebirth breathing is designed to rejuvenate and build the body by accessing prebirth chi. The belief is that diet, exercise, and special breathing techniques slow down the natural aging process from birth to death. Only prebirth breathing can reverse or slow down this aging process.

The technique is as simple as breathing. You simply reverse the natural, relaxed breath. Take a deep breath and as you inhale, pull or contract your stomach muscles in and up. Now exhale and extend these same stomach muscles down and out. This breath technique requires attention, for as soon as your attention slips, you will return to the normal, or post-birth, breathing.

To further engage the rejuvenating aspects of prebirth breathing use two words that ancients used during breathing. Because of the power of the words in conjunction with the breath, it is suggested that they first be incorporated into normal breathing. "Haah" would then be said on the inhale as the abdomen expands, and "Heng" is said as the lower abdomen contracts. Let your shoulders relax, be a bit more relaxed in your body, and let these words combine with your breath, following these steps:

1. Gently hold your belly at the tan t'ien with your hands.
2. Say "Heng" as you contract the lower abdomen. The prebirth chi will move upward from the tan t'ien into the diaphragm and be available to rejuvenate the post-birth chi in the body.
3. Inhale through your nose. The post-birth chi will fill your chest.
4. Hold your breath. The prebirth chi and post-birth chi mingle, creating a rejuvenating effect.
5. Say "Haah" as you exhale, this time through the mouth, not the nose.

In the movement the post-birth chi, considered less rejuvenating, exits on the breath, which the prebirth chi sinks to the tan t'ien. In addition, as the lower abdomen expands on the exhale, yin and yang separate.

If you like this breath exercise and want to have it be automatic, practice it. After a year or two, it will become automatic, and the prebirth chi will have accumulated in the tan t'ien ready to become a part of your ongoing health. This is the breathing practice itself.

The second part of letting the breath penetrate every part of your body is achieved by body movement and intent. Your intent can move the chi from the outside to the inside of your body and also from the inside to the outside. Intent means imagining the chi moving from outside to inside and then back again—the chi will follow your mental command.

You can also combine intent with movement. Inhale (this stretches the inner organs) and let the chi lead you into lifting and opening your arms and sending your chi from the outside to the inside. Then send the chi from the inside to the outside by combining movement and intent through your hands and arms: Exhale and let the arms relax to your sides.

Here's another approach: Place your feet shoulder width apart, relaxed legs and arms at your sides, and focus on your tan t'ien. Say the sound "Heng" and slowly raise the arms, palms facing down, fingers pointing down, and wrists limp. As your arms do this, they will climb to straight out from the shoulders. Inhale through the nose and contract the lower abdomen. Your arms are now straight out from your shoulders. Say "Haah," exhaling through your mouth, simultaneously straightening your hands at the wrists, fingers pointing out and palms facing the earth. The lower abdomen relaxes and expands back to its natural position. Allow your arms to float to the sides. Repeat as desired. This can be done in preparation for T'ai Chi practice, prior to a sitting meditation, to call your rejuvenation focus to you, or just to relax. When you've finished, rest your body in a standing position.

ESSENTIALS

Use prebirth breath when you're feeling stressed, have low energy, are waiting in line or for someone to arrive, feel depleted, still have a lot more of the day left and the day is demanding, or any time you're able to take a few minutes to renew yourself.

Staying Relaxed

The main principle for any breathing exercise is to be as relaxed as possible. Use your mind to direct the breath and chi. For example, imagine that your breath is not only going into your lungs but is also going into your shoulders, hips, and so on—any place that hurts. This is known as directing the chi. Many people actually begin to feel that the breath is going into other areas of the body as well as into the lungs.

If you're standing, imagine your legs solidly under you, filled with great strength. When you start the breath/movement, move slowly and cultivate the feeling of stability in your legs. Never go too fast, too far, or do too much. Be regular in your practice, as regular as you are with brushing your teeth. Daily movements or standing meditations create an inner environment for developing a substantial increase in your internal power. They show the body what to relax and how to relax it. The areas of the body that are tense become obvious to you: They become twitchy, achy, and generally uncomfortable. Relief comes only through pursuing mental, emotional, and physical relaxation as a part of the standing meditation.

ESSENTIALS

After you've relaxed, the body is in an open and comfortable position. At this time, chi starts freely moving throughout the body. It is this freely circulating chi that provides more energy and oxygen than is found in someone who does not avail themselves of these skills.

As you do the T'ai Chi and QiGong exercises, you will find no oxygen deficit: No shortness of breath, no trying to catch your breath, and no taking time out to get your breath in order to continue. The very nature of T'ai Chi and QiGong is that the exercise regulates oxygen consumption and keeps pace with the oxygen needs of the body. This differs from most other exercises, which put you into oxygen debt (when activated muscles demand more oxygen than is being received). T'ai Chi, when taught well, never creates this situation. Because QiGong is all about breath, it never occurs in your practice. Allow T'ai Chi to open the ligaments, strengthen the muscles, and improve your breath as it has been designed to do.

Daily Breathing Checklist

As you do your daily breathing exercises, ask yourself if you have:

- Allowed natural breath?
- Relaxed your abdomen?
- Taken a slow, deep inhale?
- Relaxed and just let the exhale go on its own?
- Remembered to do the prebirth breathing?
- Gently placed your fingers on the tan t'ien?

CHAPTER 6

Getting Started in T'ai Chi and QiGong

Before starting your T'ai Chi and QiGong practice, you can make some preparations to ensure that your practice will be more enjoyable and easier to stick to. By developing great habits, such as creating a pleasant space for these activities, inviting a friend to practice with you, playing beautiful music, and wearing comfortable clothing, your T'ai Chi and QiGong practice will be a joy in your daily life.

Timing Your Practice

Conduct your practice at the most convenient possible time. The Chinese masters probably did it in the first morning dew, but you may need a big cup of caffeine, time for a long drive to work, or help getting the kids ready for and into their day. So perhaps morning isn't for you. You do, however, have other periods during the day that may work. For example, you may have some time just before you drop into bed at night. Sometimes you watch TV, chat on the phone with a friend, share the day with your partner, or read. Instead, take some of this time to add in T'ai Chi or QiGong practice. Let it be simple—not a big deal—just a period of time to gather yourself in before you say goodbye to the day. Slide it in where it works.

Creating a Space

You may have a physical space that you can dedicate completely to T'ai Chi and QiGong, but you also may not. No matter how large or small your home, create an area dedicated to your practices so that when you enter this area your body knows it's T'ai Chi time. The following sections can help you set up this area (which may also be your living room when you're not practicing T'ai Chi or QiGong!).

The Size of Your Space

To accomplish T'ai Chi successfully, the only space requirement is a few square feet of open area. Because you can take T'ai Chi and QiGong with you wherever you go, you can do it on a lovely beach, in the park with friends, or on a mountaintop with a great view—anywhere that you can do it daily. You need only a few feet of space.

Safety

You want a space to move in that is safe—no pets or small children racing through, no smooth or slippery surfaces. You want a large enough space so you can stretch out your arms and rotate without rapping your knuckles on something. Don't do it near the tops of stairs, edges of buildings, curbs, or with uneven places underfoot. You want a space that's secure underfoot with enough space to move safely without anything you can knock over or bump into.

Air Quality

Fresh air is, of course, best, but you may not have access to quality air to breathe. There is no point in doing breath exercises if you're filling your lungs with toxins. If you live in a smoggy area, practice when the air is the clearest—this may be morning or later evening. Or find a spot in front of your air purifier or air conditioner (both of these help to clear the air). If you're in a really polluted area, get a mask to filter out many pollutants. Most air-conditioned buildings have air purification that's part of the conditioning. So if you're signing up for a QiGong class, ask whether the room is air conditioned or filled with fresh air.

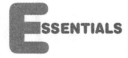

If you do have clear air, open the windows and doors or go outside in the breeze. QiGong works best with fresh, clear air to breathe and an open sky to enjoy.

Lighting

In China, there is a big emphasis on practicing T'ai Chi and QiGong in natural light. The idea is that the light carries chi, or life energy, so you want to exercise in an environment where the chi is plentiful.

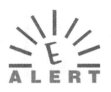

Sunlight in the very early morning is a revered time for energy-enhancing movement. Do you have a yard available or space in a room that has an abundance of natural light? Open windows allow the light and fresh air to fill your T'ai Chi and QiGong space.

If your light is artificial or limited, don't decide that T'ai Chi and QiGong won't work for you. These two activities work anywhere, at any time. There is even a story about a Chinese political prisoner who was kept in a small, dark cell but endured his ordeal by doing T'ai Chi and QiGong several times a day.

Audio-Visual Equipment

You may want your space to have a TV and VCR or DVD player as a learning aid. Move the coffee table or push back the bed to make the needed adjustments for this learning portion of your T'ai Chi and QiGong. After you've learned the sequential steps, you can move your space to somewhere that is a smoother fit.

You can also bring an audio tape deck or CD player with you, and if you find music a valuable backdrop for your practice, you can easily fit it into any nook or cranny. Some instructors also give practice support to their beginning students by providing audiotaped step-by-step instruction. This is a wonderful teaching aid and one you might ask your teacher about.

Create a musical space by choosing a tape or CD that enhances your movements.

Tape suggestions include environmental tapes, such as those of waves on a beach, bird calls, and wind blowing through pine trees. You can find environmental tapes at most record stores and some gift shops, as well. New Age music is also relaxing and is often combined with nature sounds. Classical pieces work well, too.

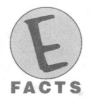

Sequoia Records has a nice selection of relaxing music. You can reach them online at ✍ *www.sequoiarecords.com* or by calling ✆ 800-524-5513. You can also reach them by mail at ✉ P. O. Box 3120, Ashland, OR 97520.

Ritual Space

Develop a familiar ritual to do just prior to your practice: drinking a cup of your favorite beverage or taking a few quiet moments to rest and relax your tensions. Sit quietly in a chair, enjoy a view, splash some cool water on your face, breathe a fragrance . . . you'll think of more ideas. Any activity like this creates a ritual space.

ESSENTIALS

Give yourself a treat that you can have only immediately prior to T'ai Chi or QiGong practice. Choose a favorite piece of music or eat a luscious piece of chocolate. How about a scent that you adore or something pleasing to wear? This technique can help convince you to drive to class or practice at home.

A Premovement Space

Simple wrist and ankle rotations can open up your joints or, as the Chinese call them, gates, and also provide a quiet preparation premovement space as you get ready to practice. See Chapter 9 for more ideas for warming up for T'ai Chi.

Privacy As a Space

Set a timer and make it clear that until the timer rings, you're in an activity that you need private time for. Linda, a second-year student with young kids, does her practice when *Rugrats* is on. It makes dinner a little later, but she enjoys that sometimes crazy time of dinner with small kids so much more if T'ai Chi precedes it!

Wear Proper Clothing

In T'ai Chi, you'll be rotating and moving your arms and legs, and your belly will be moving in and out with a free-flowing breath. This is not the time for snugly fitting clothes or for clothes made of heavy fabric. This is the time for a relaxed, comfortable fit, an easy-to-wear outfit made from a lighter-weight fabric. Stay away from denim, but T-shirts are fine. Do you have a favorite outfit for your downtime? This may be a perfect T'ai Chi or QiGong outfit—one that's especially comfy, especially relaxing. Any clothing you wear in your practice should be comfy, light, and flexible so you can move and breathe.

Proper Footwear

The shoes you choose are also important. Traditional T'ai Chi shoes look more like slippers than shoes. It is for a good reason. First and foremost, you don't want to slip, so T'ai Chi slippers have non-slip soles. You also don't want to catch one foot on the other while moving. T'ai Chi slippers fit well, but not tightly, and you want them to be flexible. You also want your shoes to be lightweight, so T'ai Chi slippers are made of cloth. T'ai Chi slippers are often basic in color—black, white, or navy blue. T'ai Chi slippers aren't generally hard to find. Catalogs, health food stores that sell clothes and shoes, yoga studios, and T'ai Chi centers are all good sources.

If you choose not to get T'ai Chi slippers, use a non-slip, lightweight, flexible shoe for your practice. I have seen many people do it barefooted and in running shoes. The latter is fine, particularly if you need the arch support they provide. If you have questions about your footwear, talk with your teacher. The shoes are one of the most important supports of your flowing movement. Without good support, the balance and confidence that come from the practice will be compromised.

Finding a Class

Taking a class is a great way to create a space for your instruction and participation. (To find an instructor for the class, read Chapter 7.) If you've paid in advance, you will be far less inclined to dodge a class, or if you must miss one, you'll probably be more inclined to take a make-up class. Hosting a class is another great way to make a committed space for attendance.

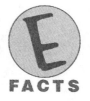

FACTS

Traditionally, T'ai Chi has been taught on a one-to-one basis: one teacher to one student. If you're in a class and feel that you're not getting enough quality attention, speak to the teacher. See if you can work out some one-to-one time before or after class. Often a bit of one-to-one is a nice support for a class environment.

If you can't take a class but want to commit to a particular time to practice, consider finding a friend to meet with at appointed times. Even if you're both pooped and want to give up the class, you'll be more likely to practice if you have to meet your friend. Two or more people create more interesting sharing and story-swapping, and you can all witness the positive changes in each other as a result of your commitment to your practice.

ESSENTIALS

A technique for creating a habit is to record your thoughts on an audiotape. Verbally complain about what you don't like, and then verbally list what you do like and the benefits you may be noticing or hoping for. Let the tape fill and at the end of six weeks, listen to it again. Alternatively, you can keep a written journal or diary.

T'ai Chi Push-Hands: Working with a Partner

T'ai Chi can be developed into Push-Hands (see Chapter 13). To do Push-Hands, both people need to know the basic T'ai Chi movements. Regular class attendance becomes a path toward a goal and a space to share your experience as you direct yourselves into T'ai Chi Push-Hands. Push-Hands can then lead to seminars in vacation spots that are located in beautiful areas where Push-Hands is also taught.

A Few Tips Before You Begin

Before you settle into a T'ai Chi class or other practice, consider tips discussed in the following sections.

Forming the Right Attitude

As you drive or walk to your T'ai Chi class, recognize that you're now entering an ancient movement, a movement that carries its own colorful, rich history that has evolved into an acceleration into better health. Be receptive. Allow the time you've committed to the teaching to be nonnegotiable.

Harmonizing Your Body and Mind

Much of what you will be learning in T'ai Chi surpasses just memorizing positions and works toward a union of your body and mind. Your mind directs your body in these consistent, sequenced, graceful motions and is constantly drawn back from its restless wanderings. This allows a type and level of attention that leads to heightened awareness: The mind is completely present in each moment. As one position flows to the next, you will develop a fine form of concentration.

This habit of blended concentration can be used in all areas of your life. Usually in our culture, the body is doing one thing—driving, running, sitting, or eating—and the mind is doing something entirely different—thinking about work, watching traffic, enjoying a concert, or carrying on a conversation. You can't truly appreciate the value of the body and mind in coordinated union until you've experienced it.

You can practice a bit before class by being mindful of, say, your walking from the car to the class door. How much of your body do you feel? Feel your legs as they propel you forward, your feet as they roll from heel to toe on the surface. Notice your breath. Think about your tan t'ien, one and one-third inches below the navel, deep in the pelvis, and use your mind to give your breath a gentle order to descend into this center. Now you're at the class door, and so on. T'ai Chi perfects this mind-body union, and the consequential growth in concentration, focus, attention, and relaxation are amazing.

Using Circular Breathing Methods

T'ai Chi and QiGong emphasize circular breathing. Imagine you're breathing in a continuous breathing pattern. Remember the tan t'ien, the energy center storage spot for chi and the spot from which each breath circles from. An inhaled breath is drawn down by the tan t'ien and goes further down into the perineum. As the inhale continues, the breath travels up the spine, into the head, and out the nose. On the exhale, the breath is exhaled out, and the golden chi floats through the front of the body. Of course, it goes into your lungs, as well!

This is the difference between breath and chi: Obviously, your breath is going into your nose and lungs to send oxygen nourishment throughout your body, and just as obviously, you exhale out your lungs and nose. The chi also goes into the nose and lungs, but being very light and permeable energy, it isn't confined to the avenues of the breath. It has its own avenues throughout the body—the meridians (chi highways throughout the body). The chi can also be directed by the mind.

ESSENTIALS

As you breathe in and out and your nose and lungs do their job of providing oxygen to the body, chi also flows into the body as you inhale, then circulates, and then exhales as you exhale. Chi travels on its own avenues and can be directed with intent.

As you practice T'ai Chi, imagine your breath (chi) running anywhere: down your arm, through your head, out your feet, moving from you to another person. It is all chi, but the breath is a terrific way to allow it to be more real. As you work with circular breathing, you'll find that the movement of the breath/chi helps you lift your arms, lengthen your back, and soften your knees. Your breath/chi will become at one with the movements, and then guess what? To direct the breath/chi, you've used your mind. So in circular breath, as described here and as it will be elaborated on in your instruction, your mind and body are functioning together (see the preceding section for more on this phenomenon).

Breathing Deeply

Even though we all think we are breathing naturally, we are actually breathing quite shallowly. Often the deepest breathing we do is when we are asleep. And if the room is not filled with fresh air, we are often just breathing out and in our carbon dioxide! So in T'ai Chi and QiGong, you will be redeveloping good, healthy, deep breathing during the day, when the sun is up and the air is fresh.

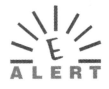

ALERT

As stress accumulates in your life, your breath responds by becoming shallower. QiGong and T'ai Chi reverse this odious trend. In order to have maximum health in your life, breath needs to fill you with oxygen and chi.

Reviewing Common Difficulties

In this section, I look at possible difficulties you may encounter in your journey into T'ai Chi and QiGong. Three areas frequently interfere with being able to benefit from these activities, but don't worry too much about them: Let the sequences come in their own time, at their own pace. Do keep the following information in mind, but don't stress about it.

Figuring Out How to Keep Your Entire Body Moving

Every movement involves the entire working body. It can sometimes be easy to forget to move both hands simultaneously and, if you're standing, to move both legs simultaneously, as well.

Learning to Have Solid and Empty Limbs

You will be learning the concept of solid and empty, having to do with your legs and arms. You are probably unaccustomed to thinking of or feeling your arms and legs this way. You can do a little preview practice by shifting the weight to one leg and letting that leg become solid. The other leg, with less weight on it, is hollow. You can do the same with your arms. Push with one as the other rests. The one you're pushing with is solid. The arm at rest is hollow.

Cultivating a Body/Mind Balance

We have created a culture in which many do no physical work. Instead, our work is mostly mental, and the body is not well used. Even for those who do physical work, the mind is often elsewhere. Whether yours is a life of a poorly used body and an active mind or a well-used body and a traveling mind, from a T'ai Chi and QiGong perspective, the basic problem is the same: The body and the mind are not unified. Even if you bike, run, or walk, your mind is still traveling. It is only in the most arduous athletics—the Tour de France, a long triathlon, or perhaps a marathon—that the mind binds with the body in a common expression.

Most people, however, don't have this type of physical endurance as a regular part of their lives. Instead, life offers continual, continuous examples of mind and body on two separate agendas. It is obvious the body gets the short end of the stick if you are sedentary, but actually both the mind and the body are cheated. When the mind and body are in the same experience, united in the same effort, there is a focus, a centeredness, an absorption in the task at hand that quiets both the mind and body. It is as if these two sides of ourselves can do things apart, but like any good partnership, they are much better together.

This cultivation of the body and mind acting in unison is fundamental in T'ai Chi and QiGong. This may be the single most important gift these two activities impart. When the mind and body act as one, the soul, spirit, or inner depth is at peace.

FACTS

Having the body and mind as one reduces mental stress and that, in turn, improves focus. The body-mind balance keeps your mind from drifting into negativity. (The mind is too busy trying to figure out tricky little T'ai Chi positions!) The body is enhanced by the presence of the mind, for then it becomes more alive and in tune with the world around it.

T'ai Chi gives the mind an opportunity to guide the body and it gives the body the ability to be more engaged and in tune when united with the mind's love of learning. The sum total is a deep quieting within. A sense of rightness in the order of things becomes more accessible. You feel in yourself and with yourself—calm, centered, present, and alert.

CHAPTER 7

Finding a Great Instructor

L earning T'ai Chi and QiGong requires little from you—no special place, time, occasion, age, clothes, equipment, previously acquired skills, predetermined beliefs, or competition. You need only you—and a very good instructor! You will need to know what to look for in an instructor, what questions to ask of him or her, and what qualities your class and facilities should have.

Selecting an Instructor According to Our Western Culture

In old China, teaching was never paid for. The master would teach a student, and the student would serve the needs of the master. This would often grow into an association that was lifelong. Throughout these decades of companionship, the transmission of T'ai Chi Ch'uan (the martial arts version of T'ai Chi) continued. Upon the master's death, the student might step into the master's place and train his own pupil(s), so that the T'ai Chi Ch'uan transmissions could continue.

When T'ai Chi Ch'uan found its way into the general public in the 1800s, this traditional style of transmission and secrecy altered into methods we are more familiar with. T'ai Chi is now taught everywhere and is one of the world's fastest-growing exercises. Unlike in old China, T'ai Chi is now generally taught in a group setting with one instructor.

T'ai Chi students in China have grown up watching adults attend to their practice morning and evening in the park. From the normality of this observed exposure, several things occur:

- T'ai Chi is accepted as a necessary and valuable part of life.
- The movements are mimicked in early childhood, and the muscle memory gets a head start.
- A sense develops of when T'ai Chi is being done well and who would be a natural teacher and guide into this world of movement, grace, health, and spiritual grounding.

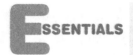

ESSENTIALS

For most people in the Western world, organic exposure to T'ai Chi isn't a part of our normal day. We read about it, see it advertised, and hear friends talk up its values. Then we decide to explore it. Its newness can be both a draw and a turnoff, but staying with it means reaping benefits that move most people beyond any reservations.

Because people usually learn of T'ai Chi from a distance and take steps to become more familiar with it, they lack the developed tools to see the difference between mediocre T'ai Chi and good T'ai Chi. Both are similar, but the mastery level is in the subtleties, the deftness, the lightness, and the ability to concentrate on the movement. When looking for a T'ai Chi teacher, you probably won't be given the chance to view teachers in an open display of their skill all performing together so you have to compare, pick, and choose your teacher in other ways.

As T'ai Chi has spread across the Western world, so have statements like, "My way is right," "I know better than other teachers," and "I make my living doing this, and I have to get students to meet my bills." These statements aren't good or bad, but they have changed the face of T'ai Chi teaching. I imagine the great masters might have some concern about T'ai Chi's and QiGong's adapted progress today. But the masters were a product of their times, as we are a product of ours.

ALERT

In ancient China, a quality teacher was more guaranteed, but it was harder to be accepted as a student. In T'ai Chi now, teachers abound, forms abound, variety abounds. This leaves the choice of a teacher, the form, the level of ancient influence, and the style of learning all very much up to you.

The exquisite mastery is now hard to find in a personal teacher, but the fact that you can learn T'ai Chi and QiGong at all outweighs any temporary loss of mastery form. With the advent of videos, T'ai Chi clubs, and worldwide travel, you can pursue your desired level of mastery of T'ai Chi and QiGong through varied sources, settle on your teacher and way of learning, and have success. You don't have to qualify to be a student!

This book shows basic Yang Style in easy-to-follow pictures and instructions. It also shows graphically how adaptive T'ai Chi is. You may find that the form suits you perfectly and that using a simple video to work out the flowing movements is a complete experience. You may, on the other hand, want to go on into learning from another teacher—a real live teacher—or other videos from other teachers.

T'ai Chi hasn't been a part of Western life for a very long time. You will need to choose your teacher by becoming informed, through trial and error, and in the end, by following your gut feeling.

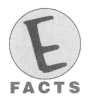

FACTS

There is much to be said for learning an art and practicing and teaching it exactly in the manner that it was taught. The reality, however, is that each successive master has altered the art to fit his own style and has sought to improve upon what he or she was taught. As a consequence, there is no one "right" way to do T'ai Chi.

Knowing What to Look For in an Instructor

A few keys to T'ai Chi and QiGong are found in the movement. For a less experienced teacher, the quality of these keys is compromised. For a good T'ai Chi teacher, they are woven into the movements such that each is subtle but obvious when you're seeking to observe it.

Relaxed Movements

Your teacher should be relaxed and calm from head to toe. It will look as if every part of his or her body is at ease. Because each movement is led by an engaged mind, the movements flow in a remarkable way. Done properly, your instructor's movements will be smooth and have a soothing effect on the observer as well as the practitioner. Because you're looking for a starter teacher who can also grow with you, you don't really want a teacher who is captivated with his or her skill and needs students to be able to demonstrate their endless prowess. You want a practitioner who does the movement out of a personal love for it and a teacher who moves in an even, slow manner—a manner that demonstrates the details of movement in a way that they are clear for your learning, not filled with the teacher's need for adulation.

Search for a teacher who has clear savvy of the continuous and circular movements. The shoulders will be relaxed and dropped, while his or her arms will hang in a relaxed manner from the shoulder joints. The elbows will point down and are never leading the movements. The balance will look as if the body weight balances on a straight line, with the root firmly positioned in only one foot at a time. This remarkably unique T'ai Chi and QiGong balancing accounts for a part of its unusual grace.

Your teacher will constantly be working to upgrade his or her personal degree of success in coordinating physically, mentally, and emotionally within the practice of the movements.

Discipline

Another key ingredient to good teaching (and good learning) is commitment and personal discipline. A teacher who understands discipline as a tool to create experiences that improve life is perfect. This is opposed to a teacher who loves discipline simply for its own sake. The first will provide teaching that allows you to become your own best teacher. The second will never let you go beyond his or her need to control your learning.

A good teacher will place a gentle, firm emphasis on breathing. QiGong is singularly devoted to this, and T'ai Chi incorporates it completely. The teacher will encourage the breathing to be natural, ever-deepening, slow, and matching the movement with both synchronized and blended skill. No T'ai Chi movement can begin to fulfill itself without proper skill.

In order to determine whether a teacher demonstrates these qualities, you will need to observe the class. This is a reasonable request, and you should not be charged a fee for viewing.

ALERT

Classes are best if taught from a starting point, so don't try to take an ongoing class that you have to fit into. At a beginning class, all the fundamentals and special terminologies are introduced and given meaning. The teacher will recognize that this early period is the most difficult and will thus express patience, enthusiasm, and sympathy.

Allowance for Self-Expression

The teacher should recognize that this is a class of individuals, and each person will have a unique way of expressing T'ai Chi and QiGong. The teacher should honor these special characteristics instead of looking for cookie-cutter lookalikes of his or her personal style.

ESSENTIALS

T'ai Chi and QiGong can be learned by anyone, but everyone who knows T'ai Chi isn't a competent teacher. Look for a flexible, adaptive instructor who understands, goes slowly, and lets small gains have the value of large gains.

Knowledge of T'ai Chi and QiGong Philosophy

Look for a teacher who has a good understanding of the knowledge and philosophy of T'ai Chi and QiGong. This can add extra pleasure to your learning. I also like a teacher who understands that T'ai Chi and QiGong are undergoing a great transition as they spread across the world, so that no one way can be considered the best method or even a standard method. When anything goes through expansion, experimentation, or exchange of opinions, an open forum of sharing and valuing is essential for this change. T'ai Chi and QiGong are changing, and new standards will evolve over time.

There should, however, be no argument on the most basic, fundamental aspects of T'ai Chi and QiGong, for these remain constant. Your teacher should have a good grasp of them, love teaching them, and recognize that variations on this theme are occurring everywhere.

Understanding Your Physical Limitations

If you have a physical problem that limits you or is of concern, share this information with your teacher. Does your teacher listen with interest? Does the teacher have an understanding of how you can best adjust to T'ai Chi? Are they willing to do a satisfying and competent adjustment? Do they suggest you check it out with your doctor first? These would all be reasonable and positive responses.

Choosing a Class Format

T'ai Chi and QiGong are solo exercises. They can be done with a group, but they don't rely on group interaction. It is always better, then, to be involved in a type of instruction that gives quality personal attention. Private instruction, if you can afford it and find an instructor who teaches this way, is best. Another option is a small class. You could get a few friends together, find a good instructor and a good location, and relax into some great T'ai Chi and QiGong. If you're in a regular-size class, make sure you get attention focused just on you. Ask questions and seek clear teaching.

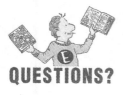

QUESTIONS?

What if no one in my area offers classes?
If you live in an area where no instructions exists, avail yourself of videos and books. Get friends to join you. In addition, take a trip to study with a teacher or get enough interested people together and hire one to come to you. Appendix 2 covers some available sources of instruction.

If your teacher seems to dislike this attempt for extra attention, the class may be too big to manage extra attention graciously. See whether the teacher has a smaller class or initiate a conversation on ways to solve the problem. If there are none, try to double up: Learn from your instructor and get a video of a master.

If a class is the best option, choose a good one. Keep the following factors in mind:

- A pleasing, well-lit space that allows plenty of space for free movement.
- A time of silence at the beginning.
- A brief but effective warm-up.
- A demonstrated review of what has been learned to date.
- The name and explanation of the new position.
- A clear demonstration of new positions with new steps taught in a uniform manner.

- Modification due to special needs made with gracious understanding.
- New steps broken into manageable pieces.
- Repetition of new steps.
- A quiet time integrating the effects of T'ai Chi or QiGong.

Verbal instruction is usually kept to a minimum, with the efficient use of cue words and the name of the position currently being done. It is best if these cues are given in a rhythm that is in the flow of the movements. A constant stream of chatter is counterproductive.

ESSENTIALS

Learning T'ai Chi and QiGong has three requirements for success:

- Correct teaching
- Personal perseverance
- Some talent for the movement

If you're in a large room, you should be able to see the instructor or class helpers easily. Each teaching person should be positioned in a way that right, left, north, south, east, and west are clear and don't require the student to change his or her position to see various aspects of the movement. This extra movement is guaranteed to add to the confusion, as it interferes with muscle memory.

Classes are usually about forty-five minutes to an hour long.

Evaluating a Potential Instructor and Class

In finding your perfect instructor, take note of the following:

- Choose your form or style (see Chapter 2).
- Observe the teacher's class.
- Note your gut reaction.
- Do you feel relaxed enough in their presence to learn from him or her?

- Is the class well planned?
- Is the class taught in a clear, non-intimidating way?
- Does the instructor listen to health concerns you may relate?
- Is the room well lit and spacious?
- Is there a time of quiet centering at the beginning of class and relaxation at the end?
- Are the fees for the class reasonable?

Adopting a Learner's Attitude

In ancient China, learning T'ai Chi or QiGong required satisfying vigorous standards that demonstrated one's abilities to respond to the demands of the discipline. Students didn't have the option of practicing the postures when they were in the mood or had the time. Instead, T'ai Chi and QiGong were a way of life. They were a work of commitment and carried all the expectations for performance and success that commitment to your career may have for you.

The instructor was a revered mentor/master who hand-selected one, perhaps two students, and endeavored to pass on his considerable wisdom to them. The structure of the teaching was rigid. This disciplined style of teaching and learning nurtured a deep and trusting relationship between the master and student. The master, like most people when they grow older, wanted to pass along the wisdom he had accumulated over decades of experience and learning. The student wanted to improve himself by meeting challenges, mastering them, and leaving his mark on the world.

To be chosen by a master teacher was desired by all students of the martial arts. It was only in gaining the master's interest that one could improve his skills. The teachings were secret and highly protected. For a talented student who lacked a bit of something and was therefore not chosen, the future had a firm limit, a wall that he would never pass through.

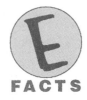

FACTS

The following are titles of mastery in martial arts:

- **Sien-sun:** Firstborn, someone who knows more than you because they were born before you
- **Lao-sze:** Old teacher, a wise and venerated person of any age
- **Chiao-sou:** College professor
- **Si-fu:** Expert, teacher, father—children who apprenticed and became a part of the teacher's life

For the chosen student, on the other hand, the sky was the limit. Now available to him was all the accumulated wisdom of a master's lineage, which he could begin to embody.

China was a culture in which one's life path was controlled by the class into which one was born. Options were further controlled by gender. (To get into the martial arts schools and temples you had to be a man.) One way to move beyond the usual class restrictions was to be accepted by a master if you had exceptional martial arts talent. You can imagine how intense the competition was. For every man chosen, thousands remained in the wings.

With all the cultural pressure and personal desire to excel, the student who was finally accepted approached this teaching as a privilege that had been bestowed—a golden opportunity. His goal became to gather enough skill that he, too, could be a master in the lineage, a credit to his master and his school, and a master of martial arts in his own right. Perhaps if he studied hard, practiced with great discipline, competed with others and won continuously, meditated, and had great spiritual growth, he would become a great master, a martial arts great master known throughout the country and remembered beyond his time. He could be a man whom others looked to over the centuries because of the great balance he had developed between martial art and gentle spiritual wisdom.

This excitement, clarity of purpose, and discipline was what was behind the student who entered his first training session. Of course he entered in reverence, honoring both the teacher and the discipline that could make such a great desirable difference in his life. This master longed to pass along his wisdom and continue the lineage. This was a personal but also a cultural goal, and it created a need to be a mentor beyond what most people experience today. They both came together, filled with hope for the outcome. They honored each other for the excellence each expressed. They respected each other and the tradition that drew them together. All this happened before the first instruction. Respect, a tremendous desire to engage in the transmission, a reverence for the lineage, and a longing for spiritual attunement generated the best possible learner's attitude.

This learner's attitude is still very much the ambiance of many T'ai Chi and QiGong classes, not because we need T'ai Chi and QiGong to alter cultural rigidity, but because it continues to carry a wealth of value. As one embodies the movements that have been passed down all these centuries, the same gift is there, the same capacity to become filled with inner peace and be in great physical shape.

ESSENTIALS

You enter a T'ai Chi or QiGong class now, in our new millennium, with a respect for all who have gone before you, all who have contributed to this skill. Go to class with the curiosity to unlock its gifts. If it is right for you, add to this the discipline to practice regularly.

T'ai Chi and QiGong will open up more each day. In this gentle unfolding lies the treasures that have made this skill so valued. If you want to know these gifts, commit to take the time each day to practice. It doesn't matter how stiff, uncomfortable, or odd the practice feels.

CHAPTER 8

How, When, and Where to Practice Regularly

It's one thing to know that something may be really good for you and another to practice it regularly. We have such busy lives, with so many habits built up, but also many resolutions to be better and healthier. Don't let T'ai Chi and QiGong become just another could-have-been, should-have-been, or would-have-been.

Seeing the Value of Practice

My friend Bernice found an unexpected way to make T'ai Chi and QiGong a part of her life and enjoy the great benefits. Several years ago, while entering an intersection, her car was hit on the passenger side. Fortunately, she didn't have a passenger in her car. Unfortunately, Bernice got banged up pretty thoroughly. After her release from the hospital, she had to heal a broken leg, a sprained ankle, a sore neck, and a cracked rib. As if this were not enough, for a month she was also unable to work, care for her kids, and enjoy her life in general.

After feeling sorry for herself for a few days (she hurt a lot!) she bucked up and decided to do something! Yoga? Too hard. Walking? Not yet. Running? Out of the question. T'ai Chi? Too painful. Her friend who taught T'ai Chi and had been pestering her for months to take it, suggested QiGong. Bernice tried it from a sitting position (not yet able to stand) and found that her modified version of QiGong helped her feel better physically and more optimistic emotionally, and it was also satisfying that in the midst of this miserable experience she was learning something new.

After about four weeks, Bernice was on her feet doing the QiGong, and after two months she was on her feet tackling T'ai Chi under her friend's guiding hand. Now a few years later, she does both QiGong and T'ai Chi each day. Actually, she wouldn't think of not doing them. They have become as much a part of her life as brushing her teeth. She is certain that without the accident she would have found many ways to put off the learning of T'ai Chi and QiGong, but why wait for a crummy life event to occur before jumping on board? Bernice's advice to you: "Start T'ai Chi and QiGong today. I am lucky to know so dramatically how healthful and healing they are. Don't just wait until you really need them. These activities improve the quality of anyone's life here, now, and forever, as long as you do them!"

Bernice had the time, the reason, and a convenient teacher. You will probably have to find the time (see Chapter 6), seek the reason, and find a teacher (see Chapter 7). Or you can wait until a life event overrides you and then think: This would be a good time to know T'ai

Chi! If, for example, Bernice had known QiGong before her accident, she could have used it to relax during the stress of the hospital experience. If she had known T'ai Chi, she feels she would have healed faster because of flexible muscles, a body well nourished by chi, and better sense of balance.

So often we wait until, like Bernice, we have to learn under pressure, or just as often, we never take the time to learn and change our life habits for the better. Perhaps one reason for this is people need six weeks before they can feel the benefits of a new physical activity. In six weeks, a lot of things can interfere with your best intentions to stay with your practice. QiGong, however, is a bit different. After just one session, you can feel the benefits of more oxygen and more chi. Feeling more energized, calmer, and healthier becomes its own reward. T'ai Chi usually requires more discipline before the rewards open up—usually four to five sessions.

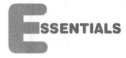
SSENTIALS

If you're poor at sticking with a program, start with QiGong. When you're ready to move into T'ai Chi, give it six weeks. By that point, you'll be feeling much better. Twelve weeks into a program and you'll notice better alertness, inner emotional balance, body tone, and overall health. Give it another six weeks and it'll be a part of your life. Actually, like Bernice, you probably won't want to consider being without it.

Making T'ai Chi and QiGong a Part of You

There is really something to be said for habits. We all have them. Some are good; some aren't. The challenge is to replace a not-so-good habit with a better one. Create a space for a habit you know is going to be beneficial, and you'll make it much easier to be impacted by this more positive choice. Each one of the ideas that follow are ways to help build a new habit and improve your pleasure in your life. You'll build positive discipline, not the finger-pointing, "you-should" discipline, but a discipline that generates more pleasure for you in your life.

Practice, Practice, Practice

Practice is always accepted as the route to progressing in learning something new: hours laboriously spent at the piano as a child or resentful repeats of spelling words or cursive writing. The problem is that practice was usually something we had to do because someone else—an authority figure—said we had to, should, would be happier if we did, and so on. As an adult, practice means just one thing—including something in your life that you've decided you want to include.

Practice allows you to make something yours. You do it only for yourself, only to make your life better, and only because you choose to.

Look Forward to It

Whenever something tedious, irritating, disappointing, tiring, and so on happens, say to yourself, "I can hardly wait to do T'ai Chi," "Thank goodness I'll be able to practice T'ai Chi tonight," "I'll sure feel better after T'ai Chi," or "When this is over, I can practice QiGong!"

Use Your Practice to Put Off a Habit

Suppose you have a habit that you want to have less of a hold on you or one you would like to break. Use T'ai Chi or QiGong to break those habits. For example: "I will have that ice cream after I finish my T'ai Chi-QiGong," "I'll have that smoke, but first I want to do T'ai Chi and QiGong," "I'll channel surf after I have enjoyed my T'ai Chi," or "I'm going to put off worrying about such-and-such while I do my QiGong."

Practice at a Low Time of the Day or Night

Most everyone has a time of day when their energy is lower than at other times. Early to mid afternoon is a common time to feel a bit flat. Some feel that way first thing in the morning. For them, a slow start on the day is essential. Still others find dusk a perfect relaxation time. Are you an insomniac? T'ai Chi or QiGong at three in the morning can not only be a great time filler, but can rebalance you energetically and make the night less unpleasantly wakeful.

Practice When Your Stomach Is Empty

It takes a lot of energy to digest food. Some people get tired after a meal and are less mentally clear, even groggy. That is a time for a walk, a quiet moment, a quick siesta, but not a great time for a practice. When your stomach is a little light, you may be a bit tired but not groggy, so this is a great time for QiGong and T'ai Chi.

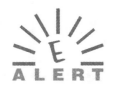

You will probably find your appetite is a little less after practice. The movement may suppress the appetite for a while, and also you're taking in energy in another way—through the air chi—and this will change your need to take it in through the food chi.

Drink a Cup of Green Tea

Green tea has a bit of caffeine. It opens the breath (and also reduces gum disease). The masters used it in the morning before meditation to stay awake.

Imagine an Invisible Practice Screen

This screen is around and surrounding your practice place. Like a window screen, it is fine enough mesh that nothing gets through that you don't want in your space. When you walk through this screen, it filters or screens out all your stress, pressures, unfinished or yet-to-be-accomplished business of the day. It filters out all feelings and thoughts that interfere with the quiet, centered pleasure of your practice. Then when you're finished, you can pick them up again as you walk out. Or just pick up the ones you want and let the others wither from lack of your interest in attending to them.

Get Rid of Aggression

If you've come to your practice feeling aggressive or competitive and you can't get into the flowing motions, take a break. Do something strenuous—running, hitting a punching bag, lift weights—and then let the T'ai Chi settle in.

Use Foot Lotion

Rub some special foot lotion on your feet. Just make sure it is all rubbed in before you start your practice so you don't slip!

Relax Your Ankles and Wrists

It can be very helpful to open the "gates" of the ankles and wrists just prior to practice. One at a time, rotate the foot and stretch it into different positions. Now do the same thing with the other ankle. Put your pointer finger between the tendons of the big and second toe. Run your finger slowly up the foot until you find an indentation prior to the rise in the bump on the top of the foot. Rub this point on both feet for a while—it opens up the upward flow of chi in the body.

Now rotate your hands, stretch the fingers, bend the hands forward and back just a bit. Shake the hands. Close the thumb against the hand. At the end of the crease you see there, rub with your pointer finger. This releases the downward flow of chi.

Practice with Someone Else

Find someone you enjoy who does T'ai Chi or QiGong. It doesn't really matter whether you're at the same level. Meet at an appointed time and at a predetermined place. Make the greeting minimal, and then get down to the business of practice. Together, you can support, encourage, and even inspire each other. You may also want to keep your goodbye simple so you can retain your T'ai Chi or QiGong space for as long as possible.

Change Your Practice Space

You can add a new dimension to your practice by going outdoors, into a different room, or into a friend's space. Each type of space will affect your practice with variety and renewed interest. Remember the most rewarding spaces and use them from time to time.

Remove Jewelry

This is especially true if they circle your neck, waist, fingers, ankles, or wrists. Jewelry can alter energy flows.

Turn Your Phones Off

Is your answering machine turned down or covered with a pillow to mute the clicking sound? Is your cell phone off? This is your time to tune out the outer world and tune into the rebalancing experience of being in your inner world and letting the maintenance of your outer world take a mini break or mini vacation. You get to be in your breath, in your movement, and in your body/mind unification.

Imagine You're Embarking on a Mini Vacation

Do you have a spot on earth that you love? Bring your five senses there. Smell it, hear it, inner-vision see it, touch it, taste it. Let your body feel what it would be like to be there. When you're ready, start your practice.

Use an Audio- or Videotape

Lie down with your eyes closed and visualize or feel yourself following along with the instructions while you're lying down, perfectly relaxed. When the audiotape is over, get up and do the movement again, this time with your body/mind together.

Watch, mimic the movements, then when the tape is over, go on with your own practice.

Relax Your Belly

Breathe while thinking of your tan t'ien (see Chapter 1). Now you can relax. No need to hold your tummy in. No present stress that creates a shortening of your breath. Just relax into your belly. Let the breath drop more and more deeply into your center. Relax into your tan t'ien and feel the fullness of the chi begin to accumulate.

Relax Your Mind

Practice after you've watched something like the wind lightly blowing leaves and let the feeling of being in light movement enter your practice. T'ai Chi is movement. Let the movement in nature inspire you, too.

Be Thankful

After you enter whatever and wherever your practice space is, say a word of quiet thanks to all those who have gone before you in T'ai Chi. Recognize before you start that you're now engaging in an ancient, loved art.

Taking T'ai Chi with You

Because you can take T'ai Chi with you, you can practice where it suits you. This is one reason for T'ai Chi's growing success. So many people who travel for a living need to exercise. With some areas of cities not safe to run in and with gyms sometimes hard to find, it is great on those overnight trips to have T'ai Chi available. Yoga requires some floor work, perhaps not to your taste in a motel or hotel room. In T'ai Chi you simply stand and move easily.

Matt, a financial planner, travels a lot. He took T'ai Chi lessons to learn how to relax as things got crazier in the stock market. He did many other forms of exercise as well, but found over time he was starting and finishing the day with T'ai Chi because it was just so convenient. As a result, he was doing T'ai Chi a lot. He started experiencing the other benefits without looking for them. His breathing improved, he wasn't getting sick from the planes' dirty air as often, his moods were more even, he felt remarkably calmer when the inevitable plane delay messed up a day of appointments, and he noticed he was more appreciative of life around him without being self-focused and self-absorbed. Matt has several T'ai Chi and QiGong videos he uses when at home and takes audiotapes when he's traveling. Then he pops an audiotape and player into his luggage, pulls it out, and lets it guide him through a session. If he's exhausted, he listens to the tape and only visualizes himself going along with it. Instead of moving his body and having his mind quiet, he moves his mind and has his body quiet.

Mixing Your Practice with Observations from Nature

The T'ai Chi Ch'uan master from the Wudang Mountain's Purple Temple was inspired by the deadly grace of the snake as it waved back and forth, tiring out the bird before its deadly strike. These great T'ai Chi masters had no TV, radio, or computers from which to be inspired by sound bites, talking heads, or the information superhighway. They experienced themselves as very much a part of nature. It was from nature that they were inspired by beauty and were fed and challenged.

They were also always aware that they could be undone by nature's wild side. No amount of martial arts skill could calm a flood, redirect an avalanche, or stave off a famine. Before nature, these skilled masters were humble learners. From their observations, they applied their interpretations, so that many positions in T'ai Chi are described with a nature metaphor. Crouching Tiger, Which Crane Spreads Its Wings, and High Pat on Horse are just three of many. Each describes the movement you will be replicating in your T'ai Chi. This naming convention provides a creative inner image for you to follow, replicates the ancient teaching style, and opens you up to the possibility of using nature as your own inspiration.

ESSENTIALS

The ancient masters that created and honed T'ai Chi took their inspiration from nature and life's tasks. It is for this reason that the positions have such vivid imaging in the title: Grasp Sparrow's Tail, Single Whip, Play Lute, and Beautiful Lady's Wrist.

Suppose you're having a bit of a problem really getting one of the postures. It feels a bit awkward and you just don't feel like you have it right. Instead of getting frustrated, take a walk in nature, down the street, in the park, or on a hillside or gaze at the sky, watch animals on leashes or at the zoo. Use whatever is available in nature. Keep in mind your posture challenge as you enjoy your walk/run/ride. As you go along, at some point you will likely notice something that fills in the missing piece for you. You will see a movement, a drifting leaf or a cloud shift position, and that will be your inspiration. You can then use your metaphor to advance in your practice.

Another great technique is to put an eye into the part of your body that seems stiff, slow to react, or not graceful enough. Suppose your back is still and stiff. Imagine you have an eye right at the base of your spine. You're not moving a stiff back. The eye is moving side to side to be able to see more. Gently let the eye imagine bringing more flexible movement to the hand. Put the eye in your palm. Let the eye see as you do your practice.

Another nature trick for a tight or painful back: When you're walking, imagine you are dragging a long tail behind you, a dinosaur tail that is heavy, muscular, and that can flick around as protection anytime you want. Or how about a peacock or fox tail? Dragging along behind you, it follows you as you turn. It swishes behind you. These images will allow you to begin to carry your back differently and in so doing reduce the amount of tension that gets backed up there.

Basic T'ai Chi and QiGong Principles

The following sections share basic principles of T'ai Chi and QiGong that allow any practice session to produce satisfactory results.

Relaxation

Take a few minutes to release a bit of the tightness in the muscles. Put your fingers to your forehead, lightly touching the skin, and let the thoughts that fill your frontal lobe just drift away.

Emptiness and Fullness

Be ready to let your body partake of the experience of emptiness and fullness that is T'ai Chi.

Evenness and Slowness

Prepare for even and slow postures. Allow a grace of movement to occur as you evenly and slowly move from one posture to the next.

Balance

As the spine is straight and vertical, practice shifting weight in your legs. This shifting of weight creates easier grace and allows a steady balance.

Rooting and Sinking

The outcome of relaxing and sinking into the positions is to root the feet, as if roots have sprung from your feet down deep into the earth. When one is rooted from the pelvis, legs, and feet, it is very difficult to become unbalanced mentally, emotionally, or physically.

Coordination and Centering

As one keeps attention focused on the tan t'ien, all movements flow from there in a complete unit. The body coordinates with the mind, the mind coordinates with the breath, the breath coordinates with the body, and so the circle goes.

Breathing and Chi

Generally one inhales breath/chi whenever the arms are pulled backward or contracted, and the exhale occurs when the arms are stretched, raised, or pushed forward. This breathing is done with the focus on the tan t'ien, and the breath sitting in the tan t'ien. Of course, the breath is in the lungs, the oxygen is in the blood, and so on, while the chi is in the tan t'ien. But if you focus on the breath doing all of it, you may find success even though this doesn't seem logical.

Meditation

There are, as a part of all T'ai Chi forms I know of, meditations. Unlike the meditation you may already be familiar with, these are standing meditations—stances one takes to quiet the mind, relax the body, and begin to promote the accumulation of chi. These are valuable to do prior to practice and also good to know during practice so that you can relax and re-relax your body as you practice your T'ai Chi. Your teacher—in person or on video—will have some stances that he or she can suggest as useful to proceed your practices. You can also use the QiGong exercises demonstrated in Chapter 12 as your standing or stance meditation.

FACTS

Meditation is a useful technique used for thousands of year to enhance one's internal skills and improve one's self-awareness in the world. Should you decide to learn traditional meditation as a part of T'ai Chi, you can find a teacher to instruct you, get a guide book, or find out what you need to know through a video.

CHAPTER 9

Warming Up for T'ai Chi

Any good exercise program should begin with warm-ups. The purpose of warming up is to literally heat the muscles and joints and increase the blood circulation. Warming up on a daily basis will improve your flexibility and balance over time, and also reduce the amount of tension that builds up in your body.

Meeting Your Model and Instructor

The photos in this chapter (and in the rest of the book) feature Fernando Raynolds, who will, in a sense, be your personal T'ai Chi and QiGong instructor. Fernando first started studying T'ai Chi more than twenty years ago when he was in college, and has been teaching for more than ten years. If you're a newcomer to T'ai Chi practices, you're in for a pleasant surprise, because this chapter is chock-full of simple, easy-to-learn warm-ups, accompanied by illustrative photos.

As you know, learning any complex physical coordination pattern (like walking, writing, or driving) takes a lot of repetition. But that is really all it takes. All you need is a model of the target behavior (as you have in these photos) and the will to repeat your efforts to duplicate the model. As an infant, you learned to walk and run and climb with parental modeling and encouragement. Learning T'ai Chi is easiest and most effective when you re-create this sort of internal learning environment. The key to practice is the attention. Five minutes of focused and interested practice brings more learning than an hour of bored and dreary repetition.

Going Through the Warm-Ups

In order to be ready for your session, warm-ups are a great idea. Your T'ai Chi and QiGong instructor, Fernando Raynolds, has put together a series of warm-up movements to prepare your body for the postures and breathing. These warm-ups are designed to get your energies moving and balanced. They will open up your joints, loosen up tight muscles, and if your energy meridians are running unevenly, help in getting the flows balanced. Do each one to your ability. If, when you do Cross Crawl, you're not marching with the opposite sides (right leg up, left arm up), but are doing same side (right leg up and right arm up) that's fine. Just keep it up, and you'll eventually cross over. This may then improve your general feeling of well-being and perhaps even your balance a bit. Your energy system is amazing, and these simple exercises go a long way toward tuning it up.

You may be able to find ways to include them in small breaks throughout your day. For example, suppose you wake up and don't feel great. You may be getting the flu. You've missed some really good sleep, eaten poorly, or you're emotional about something. Any one of these can affect your meridian flows adversely. So instead of just accepting this with resignation, you do the warm-ups—not to prepare for practice necessarily, but to feel better.

CROSS CRAWL

You start this warm-up by walking in place and touching your left hand to your right knee, right hand to left knee (see **FIGURE 9-1**). Start quite slowly; if you want, you can speed up to running in place. Do this for thirty to ninety seconds.

CROSS CRAWL WITH TWIST

Continuing to walk, increase the twist in the movement by reaching past your knee and twisting your spine. Look in the direction of your twist to bring the twist into the neck as well. As the left knee rises, twist across it to the left side and so forth (see **FIGURE 9-2**). Do this at an easy pace for thirty to ninety seconds.

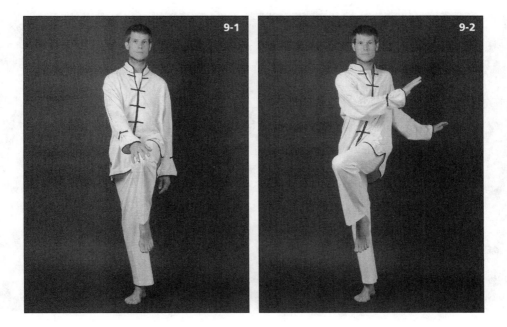

INFINITY ARMS

Continuing to walk in place, swing your arms to trace a horizontal figure eight or infinity sign (∞) in front of you. You can clasp the hands, or just keep the palms close to each other. Start drawing the X of the infinity sign going down. (See **FIGURE 9-3**.)

As one knee rises, the hands go down across it, and then rise and go down across the next knee as it rises. Do this for about thirty seconds, and then switch directions. When you switch directions, draw the X going up across the rising knee (see **FIGURE 9-4**). Do this for thirty seconds.

SHOULDER ROLLS

Roll your shoulders, alternating circling each so that as one shoulder goes up, the other goes down (see **FIGURE 9-5**). Do this about seven times, and then reverse the direction. Roll that side about seven times. When you're done, shake out your arms.

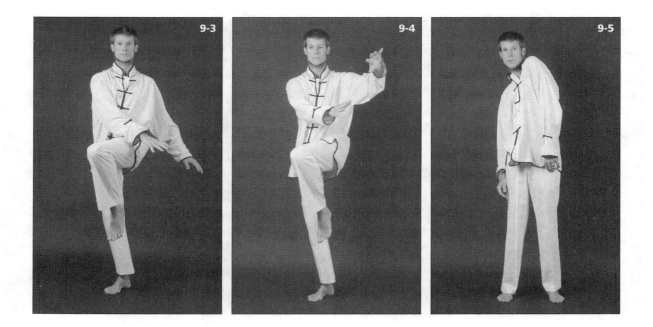

HULA PELVIS

Standing with your feet hip-width apart, put your hands on your hips and circle your hips in large circles five or six times each direction (see **FIGURE 9-6**). The weight should circle in your feet as you do this.

SEXY PELVIS

Let your arms hang and roll your pelvis as you keep your weight mostly central. Move slowly and try to make this movement smooth. Do this about seven times in each direction.

FOOT FIGURE EIGHT

This is a range-of-motion exercise for the hip joints and is also an excellent balance drill. If your balance is precarious, stand near something with which you can catch yourself. You may want to keep one hand on the back of a chair or on a wall (see **FIGURE 9-7**). If you do, try to use the wall or chair only as reassurance and keep your contact with it very light.

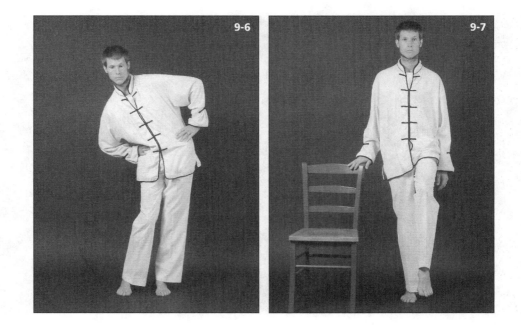

9-6

9-7

Standing on one leg with that knee a bit bent, draw a figure eight on the floor, with the middle of the figure directly beneath your hip, so that there is a circle in front of and a circle behind you (see **FIGURE 9-8**). After seven repetitions, draw the figure eight in the other direction. Repeat this on the other side. Make the eights nice and full and rounded. Notice how different the movement in the hip is from one direction to the next.

WRIST SWIRLS

Although this is a range-of-motion drill for the wrist, you can also use it as a balance drill by lifting one foot off the floor. Make sure to slightly bend the knee of the standing leg. Extend the opposite arm in front of your body and swirl the wrist first in one direction and then the other, about five times. Do this at a leisurely pace. If your flexibility is good, try bringing the foot up behind you and holding the ankle (see **FIGURE 9-9**). This will give you a nice stretch, as well. Repeat with the other arm and leg.

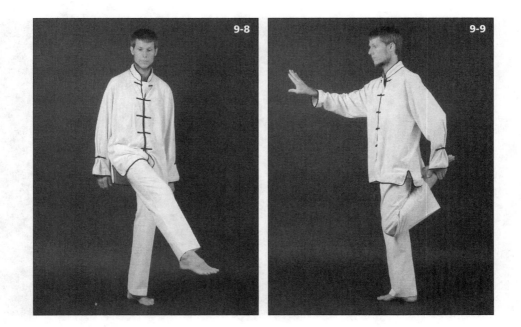

ANKLE SWIRLS

You can use this range-of-motion exercise for the ankle as a balance drill. Stand on one leg with the knee bent and lift the other foot off the ground (see **FIGURE 9-10**). Swirl the ankle seven times one in direction and seven times in the other. Do this at a leisurely pace and make the swirls as smooth as you can. If your flexibility it good, bring the knee of the swirling leg up and clasp it to the chest with both arms, getting a nice stretch.

ELBOW MASSAGE

This exercise works best with naked elbows. Start with your left palm on the front of your right elbow with your right palm near the left hip. (See **FIGURE 9-11**.)

Slide your palm around the elbow, following the fingertips over the point of the elbow. Bring the right arm up inside the left while the elbow rotates on the left palm until the right forearm points away from the body. (See **FIGURE 9-12**.)

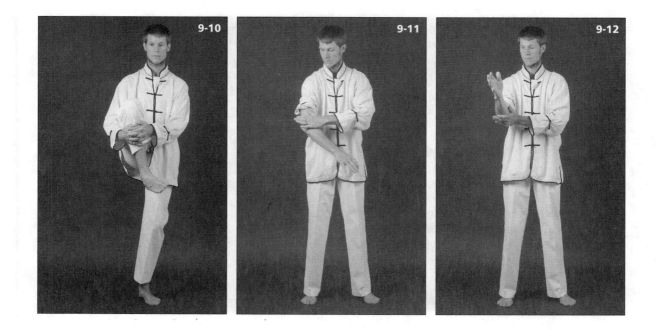

Bring your left hand up the inside the elbow and over the crease while the right palm goes back to the left hip. The movement should be smooth with both arms always moving. Keep the pressure between your hand and elbow firm, warm, and loving.

Do this seven times and then reverse. (In the reverse direction, your right arm goes down inside the left. After seven times on this side, repeat both directions.)

☯ PLIÉ

T'ai Chi borrows the plié from ballet as a wonderful warm-up for the leg and groin muscles. This is the ballet exercise in which the dancer bends and straightens the knees while standing in place.

Stand with your feet turned out from each other. The exact distance between the heels and the angle of your feet is determined by how low down you go and how flexible you are in the groin. For heel spacing, when you're at your lowest, the line of your lower leg should be vertical. (See **FIGURE 9-13**.)

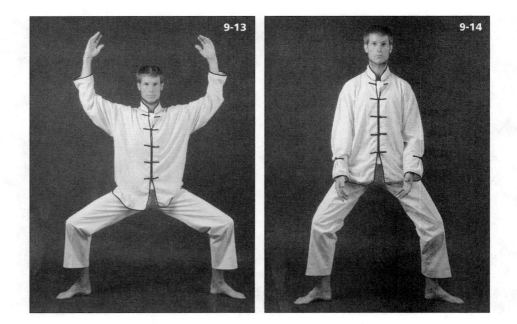

For the foot angle, keep the thigh in the same line as the foot. If you can open the groin more throughout the rise and fall of the exercise, turn your feet out a bit more to accommodate your flexibility. Don't strain. After you've established the shape of your stance, bend your knees until your thighs are no lower than horizontal. Then straighten the knees, but don't lock them and don't change the angle of your thighs at the groin. (See **FIGURE 9-14**.)

If you like, you can raise the arms as you go down and lower them as you go up. Remember to keep your body upright. It can be helpful to imagine that you're keeping your tailbone, shoulders, and the back of your head flat on a wall as you go up and down. Repeat the movement about ten times.

Stretching

The current research indicates that a maintenance level stretch should be no shorter than ten seconds, while a stretch to increase range of motion must be held for thirty seconds or more. Choose the time you spend in each position accordingly.

In stretching, it is important to be aware of the line of the stretch and to sense the muscle groups being stretched. Don't strain. Often, as you stretch one side of the body, the other side contracts a bit. In order to stretch most effectively, your attention should always be on lengthening the side of the body that's stretching. You don't want to contract the opposite side muscularly, because this can lead to compression in the tissue.

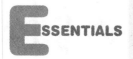

ESSENTIALS

Stretching both limbers the body and strengthens the tendons and ligaments. The wondrous body strengthens these connective tissues in response to persistent, nondamaging stress.

SIDES

Taking a wide stable stance, reach the right arm vertically, allowing the left hand to fall toward the foot. The head and torso bend to the left to allow the right side to maximally lengthen from the foot out to the fingertips (see **FIGURE 9-15**). If you go past vertical with this stretch, support the weight of the left side by putting your left palm on your leg. Repeat on the opposite side.

NECK

The neck is quite fragile, so you want to stretch it gently. Stretch your right ear up to the sky, lengthening along the line of your neck (see **FIGURE 9-16**). Do not contract the side opposite the stretch by trying to get the ear to the shoulder, because this can compress your neck! Repeat on the left side.

Hang the weight of your left arm on your right shoulder and stretch the right side again (see **FIGURE 9-17**). Repeat on the left side.

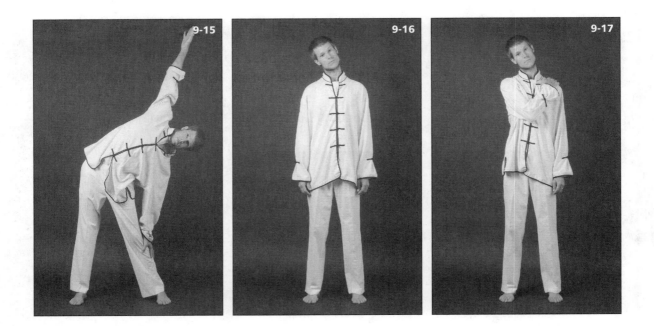

SUN SALUTATION

The essentials of the Sun Salutation, a very thorough stretching routine, are borrowed from yoga. Breathe deeply and comfortably throughout, holding each position for a minimum of ten seconds.

Stretch Up: Start with the feet together and stretch your arms above your head (see **FIGURE 9-18**). Feel the stretch from the soles of your feet to your fingertips.

Bend at Hips: Place your hands behind your lower back and bend at your hips. Don't curl your lower back—keep it straight to put the stretch in the hips and down the backs of your legs. (See **FIGURE 9-19**.)

Left Leg Back: Step the left leg back into a long lunge, using your hands flat on the ground to support the transition. Let the back of your left foot and lower leg be on the floor and the right knee deeply bent (see **FIGURE 9-20**). The first level of this stretch is with both hands on the ground, extending from your rear foot through your head and front knee. If that's comfortable, try pressing the groin more toward the front heel, making the torso more upright and putting one hand on the forward knee.

To increase the challenge of this stretch, raise first one hand and then both over your head. (See **FIGURE 9-21**.)

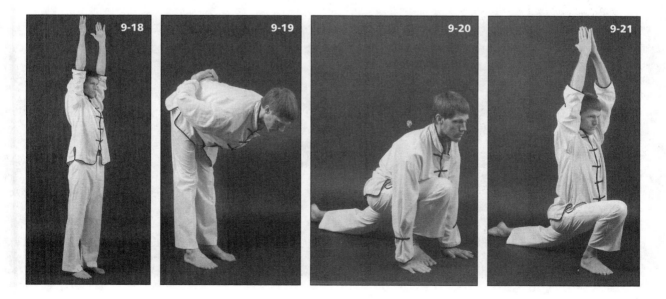

Right Leg Back: Drop both hands to the floor and step the right foot back to join the left. Rise up on the balls of your feet and arch the body up with the buttocks the highest part (see **FIGURE 9-22**). Only the hands and feet are on the ground.

Feel the stretch along the backs of your legs and Achilles tendons. Push against your arms to modulate the stretch to an intensity that's right for you. Shift the weight out of one foot and stretch the other leg more deeply. Repeat on the other side.

Diving Push-Up: With both feet back on the floor, bend your arms to bring your nose forward and down between your hands. (See **FIGURE 9-23**.)

Continue the movement, arching up through the torso until your arms are straight again and your knees are touching the ground (see **FIGURE 9-24**). The backs of your feet are on the ground, and you should feel an arching stretch through the front of the torso and chest. Continue the line of extension through the crown of your head, tucking your chin a little. This will prevent compression in the back of your neck.

Back on the Heels: Bending your knees, move your pelvis back until you're sitting on your heels. Allow the forehead to rest on the ground. Keep your arms extended in front and open the palms and stretch out

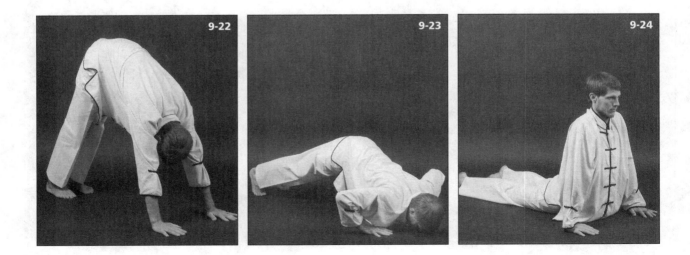

9-22   9-23   9-24

your fingers. (See **FIGURE 9-25**.) Breathe deeply and feel the expansion in your lower back.

Left Leg Forward: Come up on to your hands and knees and swing your left leg forward into a lunge. This movement is the opposite side as when you moved the left leg back into a lunge as in **FIGURE 9-20**. Keep the back of the right foot and lower leg on the floor and the left knee deeply bent. The first level of this stretch is with both hands on the ground, extending from the rear foot through the head and front knee. If that is comfortable, try pressing the groin more toward the front heel, making the torso more upright and putting one hand on the forward knee. If that is comfortable you can increase the challenge of this stretch by raising first one hand and then both over the head as in **FIGURE 9-26**.

Turn for Adductors: Keeping the weight in your left leg, turn to the side and stretch the muscles of the inside of your right leg. Your left foot can be resting on a toe or flat on the ground—you may even prefer to rest on your left knee. Use your hands on the ground to balance yourself (see **FIGURE 9-27**). Repeat on the other side.

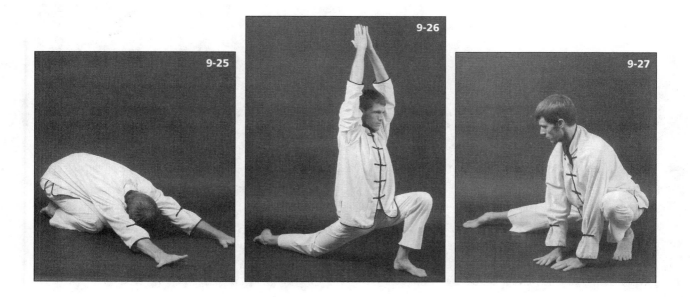

If you like, you can do both sides at once as a split (see **FIGURE 9-28**). Make sure you support yourself with your hands on the ground. However you do this stretch, be gentle and don't strain.

Hamstrings: Sinking one knee to the ground, extend your other leg out in front of you, with your heel on the ground. Straighten your leg and fold at the hip joint to stretch the hamstring muscles of the back of the leg (see **FIGURE 9-29**). Keep your spine mostly straight; don't curl your lower back. If you like, grab your foot with one hand and put your other hand on your knee.

You can increase the stretch by pulling one foot while you use the other to stabilize your body and help the bend stay in the hip joint and not in the lower back. After a minimum of ten seconds, drop your other knee to the floor and switch sides.

Bend at Hips: Bring your feet into the same line and stand up, bending once more at the hips with your hands behind the lower back (see **FIGURE 9-30**). Don't curl your lower back. Keep your back straight to put the stretch in the hips and down the backs of your legs.

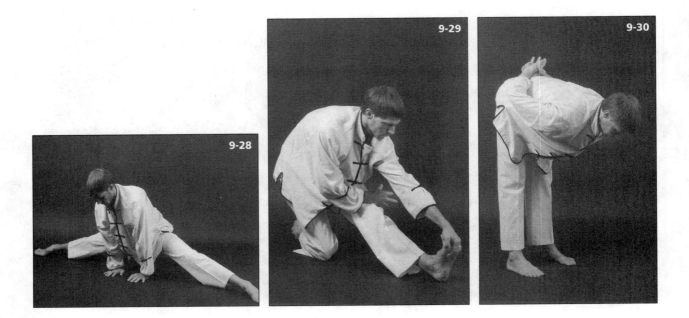

9-28

9-29

9-30

Stretch Up: Bend your knees and push through the soles of your feet to straighten up, and then stretch your arms above your head (see **FIGURE 9-31**). Feel the stretch from the soles of the feet to the fingertips.

Stretch One Side: Reach one arm a bit farther to the sky than the other, shifting your weight to the opposite side (see **FIGURE 9-32**). Repeat on the other side.

Hands Behind the Lower Back, Arching: Place your hands behind your lower back and pelvis and arch up, looking at the sky (see **FIGURE 9-33**). After ten seconds, bend your knees and push through your feet to stand erect.

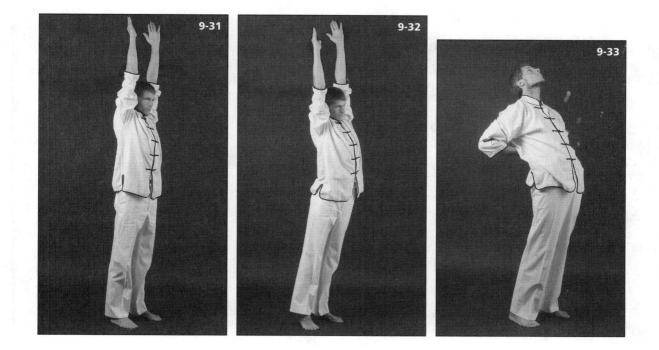

ANKLES

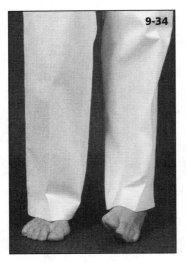

9-34

Most ankle injuries occur to the ligaments and tendons on the outside of the ankle. By stretching this side, you can strengthen the tissue. If you've had an ankle injury in the past, be gentle and use this stretch as an opportunity to more deeply feel the current condition of your ankle. Be gentle and careful.

To do the stretch, put your weight into one leg. Then, put your other foot on its outside edge (see **FIGURE 9-34**). Put weight into the ankle in a controlled fashion, giving your ankle a comfortable stress. If you want, hold onto a chair, table, or wall to further stabilize your balance.

Moving On

Shake your body a little bit now that you're done and feel the benefits of having warmed up and stretched thoroughly. Flip to Chapter 10 for more T'ai Chi exercises.

CHAPTER 10

Exploring T'ai Chi Basics

Make sure you read through this chapter and familiarize yourself with the terms and basics (relating to relaxation, posture, and sensitivity) before you try any movements beyond warm-ups. The information on stances, which is the bulk of this chapter, is also important for the proper execution of the QiGong exercises (see Chapter 12).

Mastering Some of the Basics

If you're a beginner, study and practice the basics in this section and return to them again and again as your practice deepens.

Relaxation

In T'ai Chi, the movements are performed with the maximum amount of relaxation possible while still accomplishing the intent of the movement. Muscle tone is required even to simply stand upright and breathe, so you don't want to eliminate all muscular activity. Instead you want to eliminate excess tension. The same is true in most QiGong exercises (see Chapter 12).

Correct Posture

This basic is more complicated in that there are postural requirements for each part of the body; however, the unifying theme is that you want to put the body in the shape where it can be filled with vitality. If you imagine the body as a water hose, you want to make sure the hose has no kinks so that as the water begins to flow it is not blocked. Relating to posture, this means that you want your joints to be loose and open, your posture erect, your breathing full, and your heart and mind (with your resulting facial expressions) open. In addition, you want to feel rooted to the earth: This is accomplished by keeping the joints of the legs open and springy and by opening the pelvic floor and firming the legs as if you're braced against the rocking of a ship.

Truly correct posture begins with the external requirements of precise placement. After you have a good sense of what you're trying to do, you must modify the externally dictated correct posture to truly fit your own body.

Be gentle with yourself as you learn these basic postures. They are designed to be strong and comfortable for all people, but you may need to modify them slightly to make them really work for you. This is a reason why personal instruction can be especially important (see Chapter 7 for more on finding an instructor).

Sensitivity

The correct performance of T'ai Chi and QiGong requires that you be open and attentive to your sensations. Some sensations may originate from body position or breathing, but some of the sensations arise from the flow of your chi and changes of your attention. In partner work, many subtle sensations may arise from the interaction. Because in T'ai Chi you are trying to accomplish your goals with the minimum amount of force and tension, you must be more perceptive and intelligent about the manner in which you apply your energy.

Learning the Stances

In all the stances, you are seeking to create a stable platform from the pelvis down—a platform upon which the upper body can rest. After the platform is created, you use your breath to create a sense of spacious-ness and lift in the upper body. The breath is full and deep into the lower abdomen, your shoulders rest on the rib cage, and your neck is free to allow the head to float. Your chin is slightly dropped, your tongue touches the roof of your mouth lightly (to close an energy circuit between the Conception and Governing Meridians and to help relax the lower jaw), and your head floats as if it were suspended from the crown.

Stances can be quite low, with a lot of bend in the knee, or quite high. It is important that each student seek a level at which he or she is comfortable. Lower stances are better exercise; higher stances are more nimble. Serious martial artists use lower stances for strength and flexibility training while generally sparring in higher stances. A good way to test your height is to establish a stance, shift your weight totally into one leg staying at the same level, and lift the other leg. If you can do this with good balance and control, this height is okay for you. Try it again a little lower until you run into the limit where you can no longer lift the other leg easily.

If you use a lower stance, the length will be greater. The width generally remains the same, but the length will change with how deeply you bend your knees.

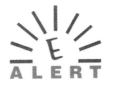

Despite some claims to the contrary, remember that T'ai Chi is not a complete physical fitness program. A more complete program would include aerobic exercise and full-body weight training.

FEET, LEGS, AND PELVIS SHAPE

This exercise is a critically important aspect of posture. It is only when you have a solid structure from the pelvis down through your feet that you can really feel comfortable and allow your energy to flow. This structure is common in many martial arts and in QiGong, as well. The general requirements of Feet, Leg, and Pelvis Shape apply to all the stances.

In the leg, the weakest point is usually the knee. As a consequence, the structural requirements of the knee dictate the way you use your legs. The knee is a hinge joint, and as with metal hinges, if the hinge is twisted as it opens and closes it will eventually break. So pay precise attention to keeping the bones of the upper and lower legs in line so that the knee is not twisted. Compare these photos: **FIGURE 10-1** is correct. In **FIGURE 10-2**, the forward knee is twisted, peeling the big toe of the forward foot off the

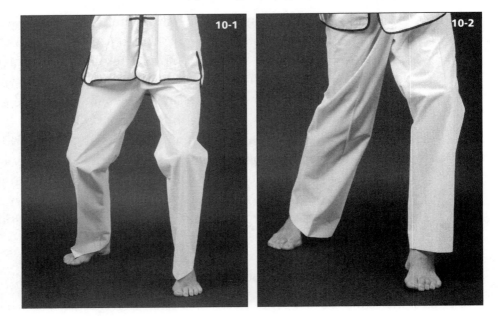

ground. To avoid this, make sure your navel points the same direction as your weighted thigh, knee, and foot. In **FIGURE 10-3**, the weight is back and your rear knee is now twisted in. Again, to prevent this, keep your navel pointed in the same direction as the weighted thigh, knee, and foot.

Protecting your knee joints requires that you spread or round your crotch so that rather than feeling as though your legs meet in the pelvis as an upside down V, you feel them meeting as an upside down U. If you do this and keep the feet at the width of the pelvis, the leg bones will be in alignment and your knees and ankles should feel comfortable.

After you're in this shape, you want to brace your legs slightly as if you're on the deck of a ship that's moving with the waves. By bracing slightly in the legs, you feel more solid and are more able to respond to whatever the future may hold. Bracing corrects the problem illustrated in **FIGURE 10-4**, where the weight is forward and the rear knee is collapsed. In this collapsed stance, the little toe will start to roll off the ground, and you'll feel weak.

In order to have a clear experience of the stance you're cultivating, I strongly encourage you to do it wrong on purpose as illustrated in **FIGURES 10-2**, **10-3**, and **10-4,** so that you have a clear experience of what you want to avoid.

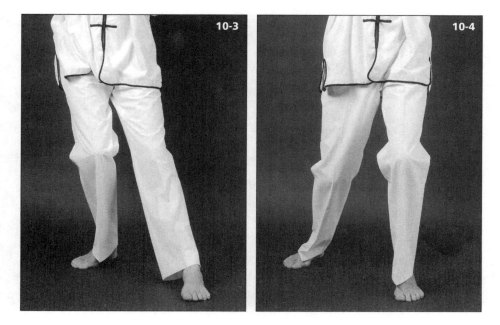

50/50 POSTURE

In the opening and closing of the form you stand in the 50/50 posture of Wu Chi (see **FIGURE 10-5**). Here the feet are parallel and hip- to shoulder-width apart.

The line of each foot is drawn from the center of the heel through the second to third toe, and width is taken between the center of the heels. Your ankle, knee, and hip joints should be slightly flexed and springy, and your crotch should be slightly rounded to bring your knees over your feet and to create a slight sense of being braced. Your posture is similar to sitting on the edge of a high stool.

70/30 POSTURE

In this posture, you have taken a step forward, maintaining your width and turning the rear foot out slightly on the heel. Your weight is 70 percent forward (hence the name), with the forward knee above the toe. Your navel points forward in the same direction as the front foot, while your rear foot is turned out at a forty-five degree angle. Your ankle, knee, and hip joints

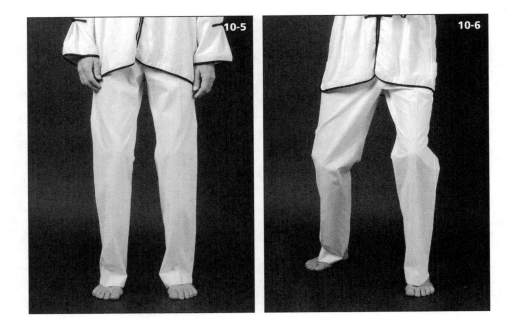

should be slightly flexed and springy, and your crotch should be slightly rounded to bring the knees over the feet and to create a slight sense of being braced. (See **FIGURE 10-6**.) In taking your step forward, you have to sit a little lower on your high stool. In more advanced practice with this posture, make sure that your heel, big toe, and little toe of each foot are on the floor and that 70 percent of your weight is in the balls of your feet.

100 PERCENT BACK

For this posture, you don't move the feet from the 70/30, but simply move the weight back above the rear foot. Although you call this 100 percent, there is still firm, flat contact between the front foot and the floor (see **FIGURE 10-7**). As you move back in order to preserve the integrity of the hinge joint knee, you mustn't twist the upper and lower legs respective to each other. As a consequence, when you're back, your navel points in the same direction as your rear foot. Your ankle, knee, and hip joints should be slightly flexed and springy, and your crotch should be slightly rounded to bring your knees over your feet and to create a slight sense of being braced.

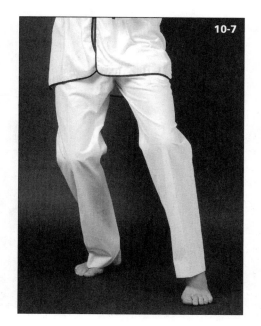

10-7

EMPTY FOOT ON HEEL

In T'ai Chi, you call a weighted foot "full" and an unweighted foot "empty" or "hollow." In this stance (see **FIGURE 10-8**), all the weight is on one foot and the heel of the empty foot lightly touches the floor. Generally this stance is used in preparation to draw back the unweighted leg. Because all the weight is in one leg, you attend to the structural requirements of that leg, assuring that the upper and lower leg aren't twisted relative to each other so that the hinge joint of the knee can remain springy. Similarly, you don't cock out the weighted hip because this tends to lock the joint, removing its springy quality. Your navel points in the same direction as your weighted foot and knee. Your empty leg is kept loose with all the joints unlocked and your knee bent. The line of your empty foot (drawn from mid-ball to mid-heel) runs a little to the outside of your weighted heel. Even in this and in the next single weighted stance, you should feel a springy sense of being braced.

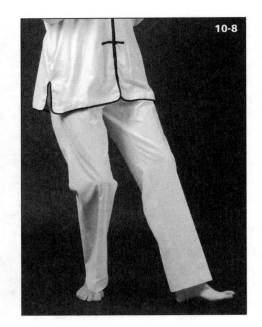

10-8

☯ EMPTY FOOT ON TOE

This stance is commonly called a "cat stance" in the martial arts and is used to free the empty foot for a kick. Because all your weight is in one leg, you first attend to the structural requirements of that leg, assuring that the upper and lower leg aren't twisted relative to each other so that the hinge joint of the knee can remain springy. Similarly, you don't cock out the weighted hip because this tends to lock the joint, removing its springy quality. Your navel points in the same direction as your weighted foot and knee. Your empty leg is kept loose with all the joints unlocked and the knee bent. The line of the empty foot (drawn from mid-ball to mid-heel) runs into the weighted heel. (See **FIGURE 10-9**.) Maintain the springy sense of being braced. Keep the line of your lower leg vertical; don't draw your empty foot back too close to the weighted foot, because this impedes the freedom of your leg to kick.

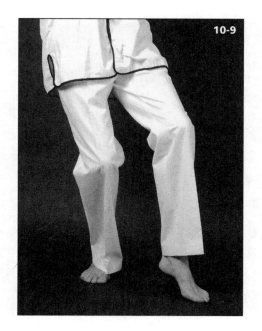

10-9

STEPPING

In T'ai Chi stepping, you want to maintain balance at all times and step lightly like a cat. In both of the following stepping drills, maintain your hip-to-shoulder width, so that you don't find yourself standing with your feet on the same line a lunging fencer might.

You start with a 70/30 posture with your weight forward. (See **FIGURE 10-10**.) In order to step, you first must turn your front foot out slightly on the heel. On rougher surfaces, this will require you to shift some of your weight back; while on smoother surfaces, you may be able to simply lift the ball of the foot and pivot out on the heel (see **FIGURE 10-11**).

Shift your weight fully into your forward foot and draw your rear foot in beside it, keeping the foot off the floor. (See **FIGURE 10-12**.)

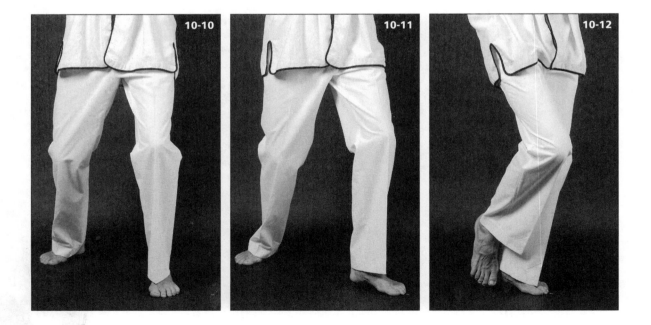

Reach out forward and a bit to the side (to re-establish width) with that foot, heel touching first, and place the full foot down without shifting your weight into it (see **FIGURE 10-13**). Now you should be in a 100 Percent Back stance. Then by pushing through your new rear leg, shift your weight 70 percent forward, and you're ready to repeat the process on the other side. (See **FIGURE 10-14**.)

Because you're stepping from one 70/30 posture into the next, you're going from a hip- to shoulder-width stance to a 100 Percent Back stance to the next 70/30. As you move through the changes of weight and position, you must continue to protect your knees by ensuring that your pelvis adjusts to keep your thigh and lower leg bones in line with your weighted leg.

When you're ready to integrate the breathing with your stepping, inhale as you draw to the center and exhale as you step and shift forward.

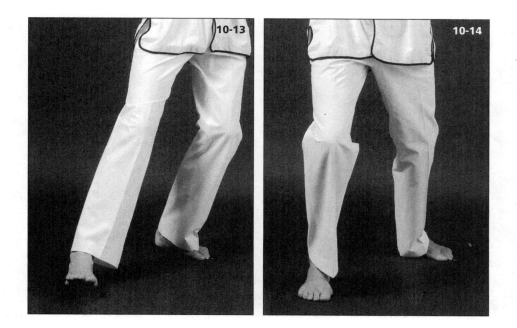

90 DEGREES STEPPING

Often, you need to adjust your stance to face a new challenge. This step teaches you how to step in strongly at 90 degrees. Starting with a 70/30 Posture facing north with your weight forward on the left leg (see **FIGURE 10-15**), you shift fully into your forward leg, drawing your right leg in beside your left (see **FIGURE 10-16**).

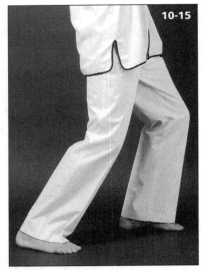

Turning the gaze 90 degrees to east, you step east and to the side (for width) on your heel, rolling your foot down flat with no weight (see **FIGURE 10-17**). Then, by pushing out of the heel of your new rear foot, shift the weight 70 percent forward. As you do so, the Foot, Leg, and Pelvis requirement has you turn the rear foot in on your heel (see **FIGURE 10-18**). Pay attention at this point to ensure that you don't turn in on your toe, nor that you collapse your rear knee. If you have a tendency to want to pivot on the ball of

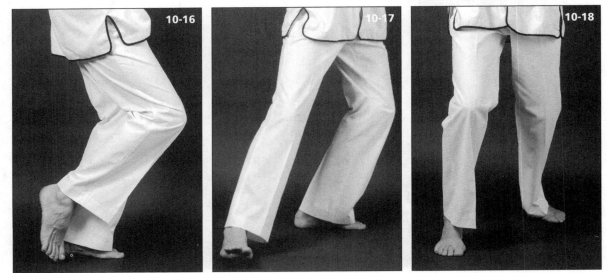

your foot, usually you're stepping too narrowly. If you draw a line forward from the center of your rear heel that's parallel with the line of your forward foot, the lines should be hip- to shoulder-width apart.

The mechanics of the 90-degree stepping drill can be adopted to a 135-degree stepping drill for a more advanced exercise.

Practicing the Hand and Arm Postures

The requirements of hand and arm postures reflect the two concerns of energy flow and effective body mechanics.

 BEAUTIFUL LADY'S WRIST

Beautiful Lady's Wrist refers to a postural requirement emphasized by Cheng Man-Ching that is often not stressed in other schools of T'ai Chi. This term simply refers to holding your wrist in an open position so that your energy is free to flow into your palms (see **FIGURE 10-19**). The wrist is not bent in any way. More advanced manifestations of this quality are no obstructions at the wrist and energy streaming through the wrist.

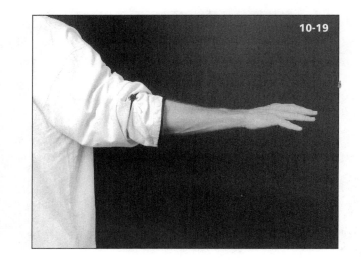

10-19

PALMS RESTING ON PILLOW OF AIR

When one or both arms are at your sides, they must remain alive and not become limp. An alive arm at rest has a slight forward curve at the elbow and wrist, almost as if the arm is resting on an updraft of air. This is called having the palm resting on a pillow of air (see **FIGURE 10-20**). Generally, the martial meaning of this posture is pulling down and back.

 SHOULDER DOWN TO ELBOW, UP TO WRIST

This is a general rule for arm structure in which you keep the elbows down and weighted in order to ensure that the shoulder blades remain attached to the latissimus dorsi muscles (shoulder muscles of the back) and thus to the rib cage and your body as a whole. Unless your arm is raised so high that your elbow must be higher than the shoulder, the line of the arm goes down from shoulder to elbow. And unless your hand is so low that your wrist must be lower than the elbow, the line then goes up to the wrist.

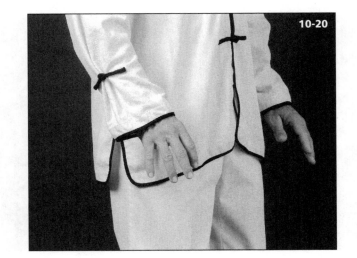

10-20

HOLDING THE BALL

This posture is often used in T'ai Chi as a transitional movement and is a good opportunity to reconnect with your sense of energy between your palms. The energy ball that's held is generally the size of a large beach ball. If vertical, the lower hand is at the level of the navel while the upper hand is at the level of the collarbones. (See **FIGURE 10-21**.) This posture has myriad defensive and offensive applications.

WARD OFF

In this posture, either or both arms are in an arc in front of your body with your palm facing the center line at about the level of the base of the sternum (see **FIGURE 10-22**). Your arm(s) follow the "Shoulder Down to Elbow, up to Wrist" rule. This posture is used as an extra layer of protection between you andthe incoming energy. It can also be used as a posture to attack with your forearm.

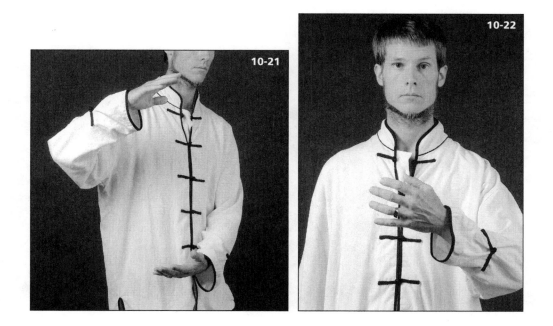

10-21

10-22

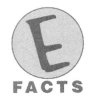

FACTS

Peng or Ward Off is a central energy in T'ai Chi and should be present in all of your movements. Think of it as the energy inside an inflated balloon. You literally expand your body into a more resilient structure. Having braced your legs, you then extend your arms and the torso with Peng energy to create an even more stable and resilient structure.

TWO-HANDED PUSH

In this posture you position yourself as if you were pushing a van out of a ditch (see **FIGURE 10-23**). Your arms follow the Shoulder Down to Elbow up to Wrist rule, and your palms face away from your body as wide apart as your shoulders, with your fingertips no higher than your shoulders. You use Beautiful Lady's Wrist, although in application, your hands would conform with the object being pushed.

ONE-HANDED PUSH

This posture is the same as the Two-Handed Push method except that you use only one hand. As a consequence, the pushing hand must move closer to the midline in order to maintain power (see **FIGURE 10-24**). The first knuckle of the thumb tends to be on the midline.

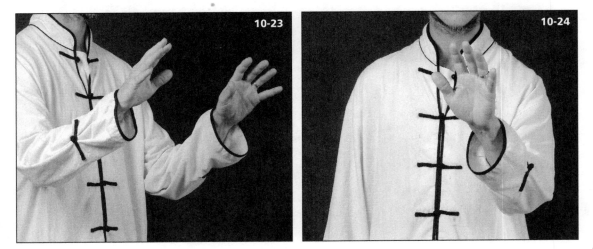

10-23   10-24

HOOK HAND

This is a signature hand position for T'ai Chi. Here, the tips of the fingers all touch the tip of the thumb. The hand then hangs lightly from the wrist. (See **FIGURE 10-25**.) This consolidates the strength of the fingers in to a single "beak," which can be used to strike small targets like eyeballs. In some martial applications, this hand position is also used to signify a grab with that hand.

FIST

The T'ai Chi Fist is held lightly, with the fingers closed and the thumb curled down and over them (see **FIGURE 10-26**). There is a little space within the fist. If you imagine you've captured a tiny fairy, don't squeeze and crush the fairy. In a martial application, however, the fist is tightened just before the point of impact.

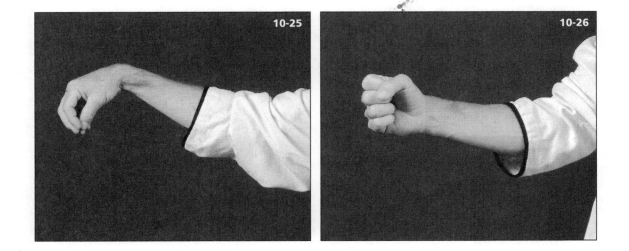

10-25

10-26

Understanding Form Instructions

The T'ai Chi series of movements (or form) presented here is called the Yang Style short form, abridged by Cheng Man-Ching. Professor Cheng (following the Chinese pattern, the surname is first) was a highly respected T'ai Chi master, as well as a master of calligraphy, painting, and of Traditional Chinese Medicine (TCM). He was one of the first T'ai Chi masters to teach T'ai Chi to non-Chinese in the United States. Finding Americans to be a rather impatient people, he shortened the form to fit more easily with our hurried lifestyles. He took the traditional Yang Style, which is said to have 108 movements, and removed the repetitions to create his shortened form. The first portion of this form, about one third of the full length, is presented here. This portion is a manageable chunk to learn from a book and is also almost identical with the first portion of the longer, more traditional Yang form. As a consequence, if you start learning T'ai Chi from this book and later choose to study more, you will be able to build on this material with a class or video on either Professor Cheng's form or the traditional Yang Style long form.

CHAPTER 11
Advanced T'ai Chi

The original purpose of T'ai Chi was to train the body and mind for self-defense, whereas QiGong practice involves energy exercises that don't necessarily have a martial arts component. After you have a feel for a given movement, refer to Chapter 18 to more deeply understand its purpose.

Getting a Few Reminders Before You Begin

Keep the following postural reminders in the forefront of your mind as you advance in your T'ai Chi practice:

- Keep your tongue lightly touching the roof of your mouth to close the circuit between the Conception and Governing meridians.
- Inhale and exhale deeply into your abdomen through your nose.
- Keep your spine vertical; don't lean to the side or forward or back.
- Feel and relax your entire body.
- Maintain a sense of connection with the energy of the earth through the balls of your feet.
- Allow your head to float as if suspended from above.
- Keep Beautiful Lady's Wrist, Shoulder Down to Elbow up to Wrist, and Feet, Legs, and Pelvis Shape.
- When extending your arms, don't extend past a vertical line up from your forward knee.
- When reaching an arm back behind, don't open the front of your shoulder socket by taking your upper arm back too far.
- Remember to counterbalance your movements.
- Move slowly and purposefully without breaks, pauses, or accelerations.
- Move your whole body as one unit with the movement originating from your legs and engaging the core, deep muscles of your abdomen in the tan t'ien.

Recognize that the whole body should start and stop at the same time, moving everything at once. Due to the limitations of a written narrative, it may seem as though your right arm is moved first and then your left. The narrative is broken up by movement and by breath. All movements described with a given breath, however, should be done as a single flow.

Although this chapter includes the breathing pattern to give you a sense of the flow, ignore your breath at first and concentrate on getting the movements down. After you have a good sense of the movements, add the breath cycle. As you add your breathing, don't follow the suggested pattern rigidly. In movements such as Single Whip; White Crane

Spreads Wings; and Deflect Downward, Parry and Punch; the exact transition point for inhale to exhale is quite subjective.

Learning the Advanced Movements

To learn these movements from the book, you may want to either have someone read you the instructions or else make an audiotape of them for yourself. It is almost impossible to learn these if you have to stop every few moments to read what to do next. The photos are shot from an angle designed to show you all four limbs clearly, so pay attention to the written instructions to be clear about the direction faced. Sometimes, you may need to read through the instructions and study the photos a couple of times before you understand them. Be patient. This chapter usually requires from eight to twelve class hours, so don't expect to master this material too rapidly.

For each movement, I give its stance type and the direction faced at the completion of the movement. When learning, after completing a movement, check your stance from your feet up, making sure that you're following the requirements of the basics and that your body is relaxed and comfortable. After you know the movements, they should flow one into the next at an easy pace with no break.

Learning a movement is based on repetition, so it can be helpful to repeat part of a movement or several movements in a series in a more rapid and cursory way. This clarifies the pattern of movement in your mind so that you can go through it more slowly with greater attention to detail.

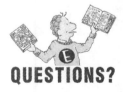

QUESTIONS?

Are there "belts" in T'ai Chi?
Not generally, but according to instructor Gene Burnett, there are four interconnected levels of work in T'ai Chi:

The bone level: Fundamental principles.
The muscle level: Relaxation.
The energy level: A deeper energetic connection.
The spiritual level: Surrendering ego-control and identification.

PREPARATION, WU CHI

(Stance type/direction: 50/50 N.) Stand in your Wu Chi (as described in Chapter 12) for long enough to settle your mind and clear the mental and emotional space to proceed (see **FIGURE 11-1**).

 BEGINNING, LIFTING HANDS

(Stance type/direction: 50/50 N.) Exhale and allow your shoulders to become a little concave, initiating forward momentum in your arms. Inhale and support that momentum by raising your arms up, drawing energy up from the earth. The palms droop down at your wrists (as if your arms are moving through water) and rise until they are slightly lower than your shoulders (see **FIGURE 11-2**). Exhale and straighten your wrists, extending the energy out through your fingertips.

As air pressure in your lungs decreases, allow your elbows to settle downward, bringing your wrists back toward your shoulders in a Begging Dog posture (see **FIGURE 11-3**). Inhale and straighten your wrists, fingers to the sky, drawing in energy from the heavens. Exhale and settle the energy down the right and left sides of your body with your hands

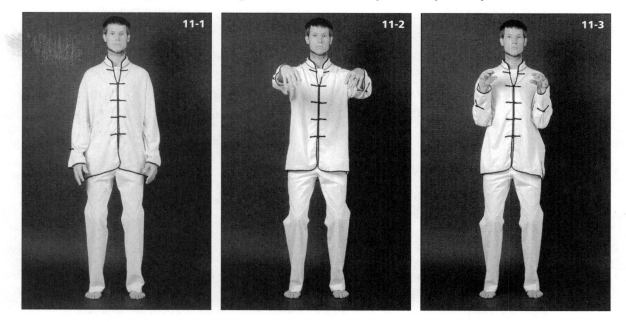

going down to your sides to Rest on a Pillow of Air. The movement of the arms should be subtly counterbalanced by bending your knees more and sitting with your pelvis as your arms go up and out and straightening slightly as your hands come close to your body.

GRASP SPARROW'S TAIL, WARD OFF LEFT

(Stance type/direction: 70/30 N.) In this movement, your legs essentially follow the requirements of the 90 Degrees Stepping as described in Chapter 10. Inhale as you shift your weight into your left foot and turn on your right heel to the right. Your arms flow with the momentum of the turn, creating a vertical ball on your right side with the right hand high, left hand low (see **FIGURE 11-4**).

Exhale as you bring your left foot into the center and reach out northward and to the side. Touch your heel first and then roll into your foot. As you shift into your left foot and execute your arm movements, pivot your right foot in on the heel to forty-five degrees. Settle your right arm down to Rest on a Pillow of Air while your left arm expands forward into a Ward Off Left with the palm facing the center of your chest at about the level of the bottom of your breast bone (see **FIGURE 11-5**).

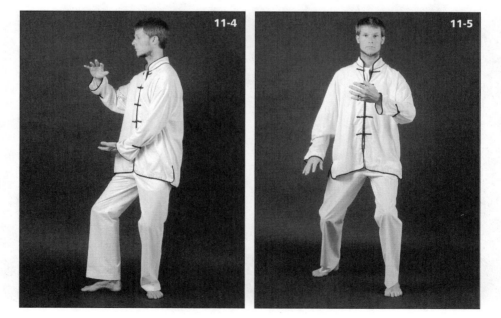

11-4

11-5

GRASP SPARROW'S TAIL, WARD OFF RIGHT

(Stance type/direction: 70/30 E.) In this movement, your legs essentially follow the requirements of the 90 Degrees Stepping as described in Chapter 10. Inhale as you draw your right foot into the center and scoop your right hand past your groin, turning your left palm down to hold a vertical ball, your right hand below (see **FIGURE 11-6**).

Step east, reestablishing the width of your stance. The heel of your right foot touches first, and then you roll your foot down. Exhale as you push and roll the ball between your hands to the front, ending up with your palms facing each other horizontally as if holding a soccer ball (see **FIGURE 11-7**). Your left hand is closer to your body. Make sure that your left foot pivoted in forty-five degrees on your heel and that you stepped with adequate width for your stance.

 ## GRASP SPARROW'S TAIL, ROLLBACK

(Stance type/direction: 100 Percent Back in left NE.) In this movement, your feet don't move. Inhale, twisting your torso a few

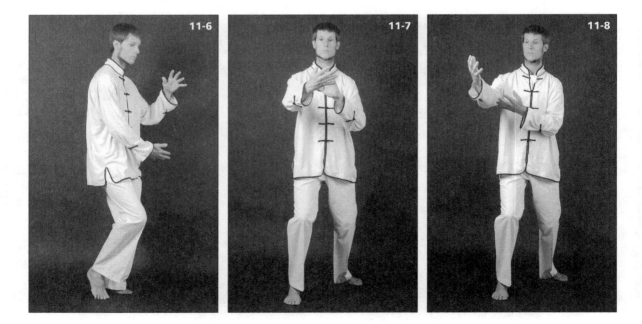

degrees to the right. Your right arm extends a bit to the corner while your left palm turns to face your right elbow (see **FIGURE 11-8**).

Exhale as you shift the weight into your left foot, remembering to allow your pelvis to turn in order to preserve your Feet, Legs, and Pelvis Shape. You end up holding a ball almost horizontally by your left hip with your right hand a little higher than your left (see **FIGURE 11-9**).

GRASP SPARROW'S TAIL, PRESS

(Stance type/direction: 70/30 E.) In this movement, your feet don't move. Inhale, allowing your left arm to continue its swing upwards and northward, and fold it at your elbow so that your fingers are by the ear. Your right hand turns palm up, continuing to hold the ball (see **FIGURE 11-10**).

Exhale, and then push and compress the ball until your left palm presses against your right with your left palm closer to your body, hands on the midline at mid-chest level. The hollow of your left palm receives the muscle of the thumb of the right palm (see **FIGURE 11-11**).

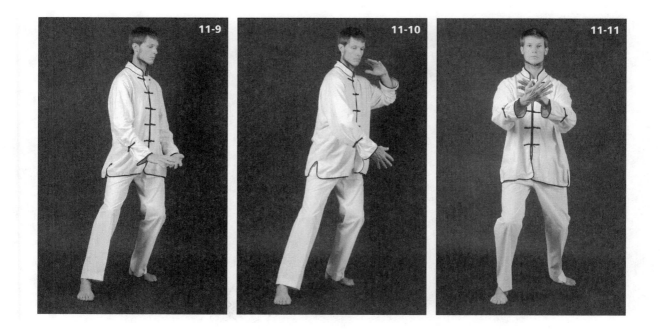

GRASP SPARROW'S TAIL, PUSH

(Stance type/direction: 70/30 E.) In this movement, the feet don't move. Inhale as your left hand presses through the right, with your hands separating to shoulder width and withdrawing to just in front of your shoulders, palm facing away as you shift 100 Percent Back into your left leg. Don't draw your arms so far back that you feel exposed or that you tighten across your chest. Because you're shifting into your rear leg, your pelvis will rotate slightly left to keep your knee alignment. Your intention and your hands and torso, however, should remain facing east (see **FIGURE 11-12**).

Exhale as you shift your weight forward and push your hands away at the same level. End in a Two-Handed Push position in a 70/30 stance (see **FIGURE 11-13**).

SINGLE WHIP

(Stance type/direction: 70/30 W.) In this movement, you turn 180 degrees around. The last part of the foot movement is a 90 Degrees Step. Inhale as you shift back into your left leg, allowing your pelvis to turn to

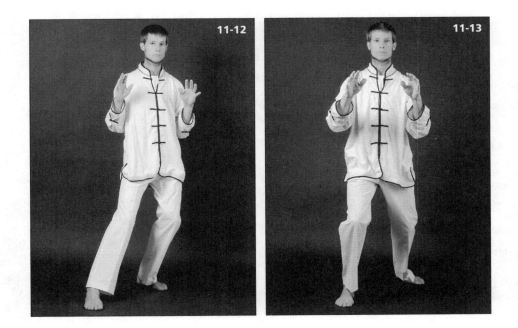

the left. Your arms extend as if your fingertips remained where they were at the end of Push. Continue inhaling as you turn to the left, carrying your arms in alignment with your torso so that they end up to the north. Your right foot turns north on your heel (see **FIGURE 11-14**).

Exhale and compress and draw into your right leg. As the weight comes out of the left and your leg is drawn in, allow your left foot to pivot on the ball. Your left arm drops, palm up, near your right hip. Your right hand makes a Hook Hand and your elbow drops, folding your arm to bring your right hand over your left palm. Inhale and counterbalance doing the 90 Degrees Step with your left hand and to the west by extending your hooked right hand out to the north-northwest (see **FIGURE 11-15**).

Exhale as you bring your left arm up from your left hip to in front of your left shoulder in a protective sweep with your palm facing your body. Finish by turning your left palm away and extending your left arm into a One-Handed Push as you complete the pivot of your right foot on your heel to forty-five degrees (see **FIGURE 11-16**).

More advanced: After your left foot is placed, relax your right arm and sink your elbow. Then counterbalance your left hand going into the Push by bringing the right hook arm a little to the right rear.

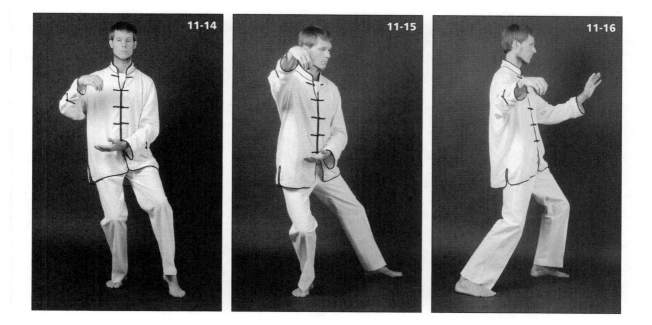

LIFT HANDS, OPEN/CLOSE

(Stance type/direction: Empty right foot on heel NW.) Inhale, open the hook, and spread your arms open in a welcoming embrace facing forward by dropping your elbows as you shift 100 Percent Back into the left leg. Pay attention to the structural requirements of the left leg and don't twist your joints (see **FIGURE 11-17**).

Exhale and close your arms to the midline. Your arms move slightly down and then back up to engage the shoulder muscles of your back (the latissimus dorsi). The left palm ends facing your right elbow with a few inches of space between. As the arms close, your right foot comes into the center and then out northwest on your heel (see **FIGURE 11-18**).

 ## SHOULDER STROKE

(Stance type/direction: NW.) Inhale and Roll Back to the left side, ending with a horizontal ball near your left hip with your right hand a little higher. At the same time, draw your right foot back to just behind your left ankle (see **FIGURE 11-19**).

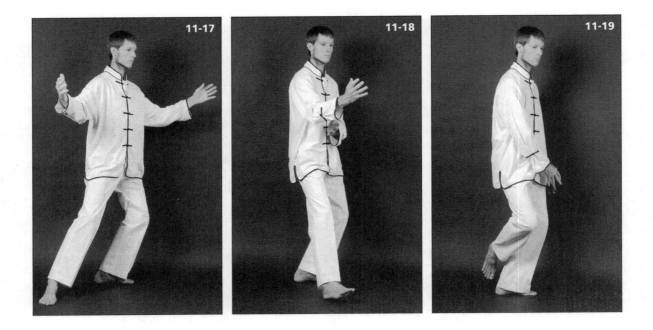

11-17 11-18 11-19

Replace your right foot and exhale as you shift eighty degrees of your weight forward. Your right arm remains mostly stationary and is carried by your torso. Your left arm twists palm down and rises until the first knuckle of your thumb is at the midline. The left arm is Shoulder Down to Elbow up to Wrist and your right arm is in a stronger arc with your palm up to the rear. Both arms are close in to the front of your body. Make sure you have good leg and pelvis structure and that your knees aren't twisted (see **FIGURE 11-20**). Your head should be turned a little to the right so that you can look over your right shoulder.

WHITE CRANE SPREADS WINGS

(Stance type/direction: Empty left foot on toe, W-NW.) Inhale and shift your weight more into your right leg as your left hand moves down your midline and your right moves up. They pass each other with your left hand closer to the body (see **FIGURE 11-21**).

Exhale as at the solar plexus (the area of the belly just below the sternum) your right forearm starts rolling with your palm facing the body, then down, then away. Your left arm can maintain its angle, but goes left from the

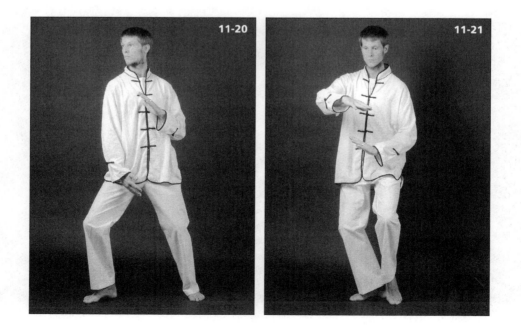

center line as it passes the tan t'ien. Your left foot comes in to the center and reaches out on your toe. As your foot moves in, your body is released to turn a little more to the right, and you conclude with your left hand on the Pillow of Air and the right arm in an oblique salute with the back of the palm facing the temple, about a fist distance away. This is one of the few postures where your (right) elbow is higher than your shoulder (see **FIGURE 11-22**).

BRUSH KNEE AND TWIST

(Stance type/direction: 70/30 W.) Inhale as you drop your right elbow and raise your left hand as your left arm moves across your body to the right so that you're holding a diagonal ball on your right with your left hand high (see **FIGURE 11-23**).

Drop your left arm, palm down, and raise your right arm to the north, palm up. Use the counterbalance of your arm to allow you to bring your left foot into the center (see **FIGURE 11-24**), and then step west (with enough width).

After your heel touches, fold your arm at your elbow, bringing your hand palm down near your right shoulder. Exhale, shift into your left leg,

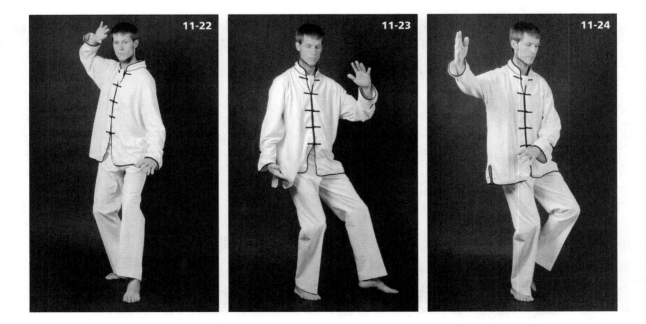

sweep your left arm across to the left with your fingertips just above the knees, and execute a Single-Handed Push with your right hand, the first knuckle of the thumb ending up on the centerline, your fingertips just lower than your shoulder (see **FIGURE 11-25**).

☯ PLAY LUTE

(Stance type/direction: Empty left foot on heel N-NW.) Inhale, shifting your weight fully into your left foot, drawing your right knee in beside your left and reaching forward a bit with your right hand as your left arm settles downward, with your palm facing your body (see **FIGURE 11-26**).

Step your right foot back down facing northwest. Exhale as you shift back and allow your pelvis to turn a bit to the right. Use that momentum to raise your left leg a little forward onto your heel and your left arm forward and up with your palm on the midline pointing to the upper right. Draw your right arm back so that your right palm faces your left elbow with three to four inches between (see **FIGURE 11-27**).

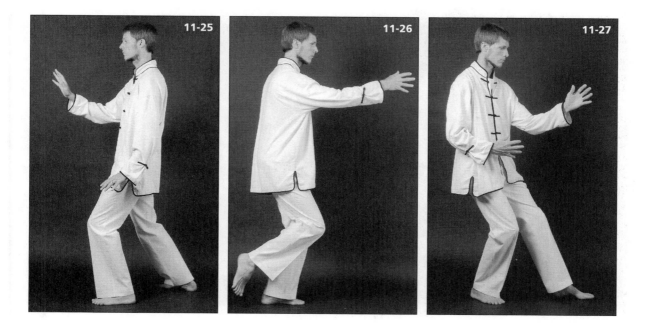

BRUSH KNEE AND TWIST

(Stance type/direction: 70/30 W.) Inhale as you drop your right elbow and move your left hand across your body to the right so that you're holding a diagonal ball with your left hand high (see **FIGURE 11-28**).

Drop your left arm, palm down, and raise your right arm to the north, palm up. Use the counterbalance of your arm to allow you to bring your left foot into the center and then step west (with enough width). After your heel touches, fold your arm at your elbow, bringing your hand palm down near your right shoulder. Exhale, shift into your left leg, sweep your left arm across to the left with your fingertips just above the knees, and execute a Single-Handed Push with your right hand, the first knuckle of the thumb ending up on the centerline, your fingertips just lower than your shoulder (see **FIGURE 11-29**).

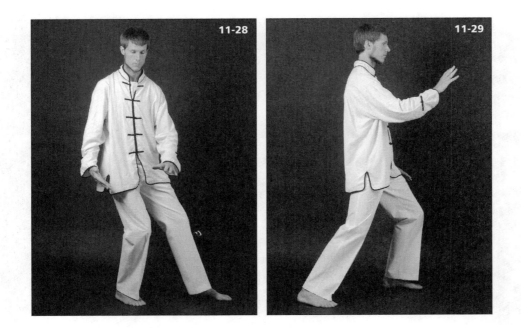

STEP FORWARD, DEFLECT DOWNWARD, PARRY AND PUNCH

(Stance type/direction: 70/30 W.) This movement incorporates a forward step first with your right leg, then your left. Inhale as you turn your left foot out slightly to the left with your whole body. Drop your right hand to your left side so that you hold a horizontal ball over your left thigh and form a fist with your right hand (see **FIGURE 11-30**).

Counterbalance with your arms circling up to the left (south), your right fist near your left armpit, as you draw your right foot into the center. Begin your exhale and step your right foot forward and to the side with your foot pointed northwest (see **FIGURE 11-31**).

Your left arm folds at your elbow, bringing your hand near your left ear, and your right fist arcs forward as a back Fist Strike as you shift into your right leg (see **FIGURE 11-32**).

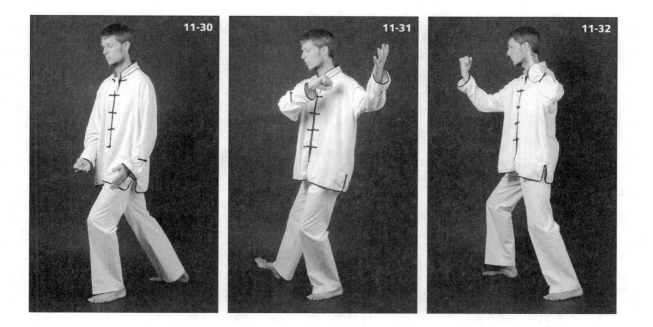

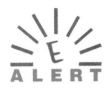

ALERT

Whenever I'm dissatisfied with my progress in T'ai Chi, I've found that I have simply been going through the motions in some area of my practice. To progress, I must improve the quality of my practice. In T'ai Chi, as in much of the rest of your life, quality matters more than quantity.

Inhale as you shift your weight fully into your right foot, drawing your left foot into the center and reaching it forward and to the side. Your right fist continues its arc to withdraw to your right hip, and your left arm reaches forward on the midline. The movement and timing of your arms counterbalance each other here (see **FIGURE 11-33**).

Exhaling, draw your left hand back on your left side of the midline and punch forward with your right (the whole shoulder girdle turns) as you shift into your left leg, pelvis turning into a 70/30 stance. The fist finishes vertical, just right of the midline, at solar plexus height (see **FIGURE 11-34**).

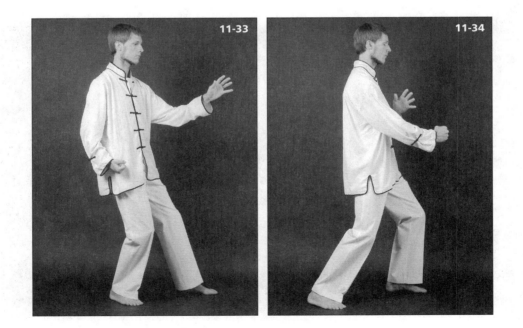

APPARENT CLOSE UP OR WITHDRAW AND PUSH

(Stance type/direction: 70/30 W.) In this movement, your feet don't move as you shift your weight back and then forward. Inhaling, extend your right arm a bit to the left corner, opening your fist and reaching under your right elbow with your left palm up (see **FIGURE 11-35**).

Shift your weight 100 Percent Back into your right leg, drawing your right arm back across the top of your left wrist. Form a horizontal ball at solar plexus height to the right side (see **FIGURE 11-36**).

Exhaling, shift your weight back into a 70/30 stance and execute a Two-Handed Push (see **FIGURE 11-37**).

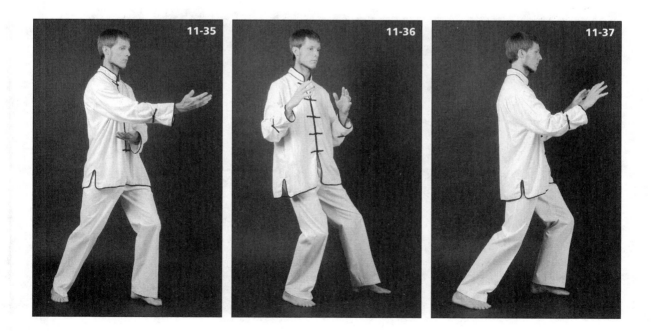

11-35 11-36 11-37

CROSS HANDS

(Stance type/direction: 100 percent in left, feet parallel N.) Inhale as you shift your weight back. Release the ball of your left foot and turn to the north on your left heel. Your arms are carried with your body, rising slightly so that your fingers are at eye level (see **FIGURE 11-38**).

After your left foot is pointed north, sink into it and drop your arms down in twin arcs until they cross in front of your groin, palms facing away, your left arm closer to your body. As your right leg empties, your foot is free to pivot inward on the ball. Draw your right foot into the center (with your crossed arms, slightly, as well—see **FIGURE 11-39**) and exhale as you place your right foot down hip- to shoulder-width and parallel with your left foot. At the same time, your arms rise in an upward diagonal to your shoulder height. Your arms are still crossed a little below your wrists (see **FIGURE 11-40**).

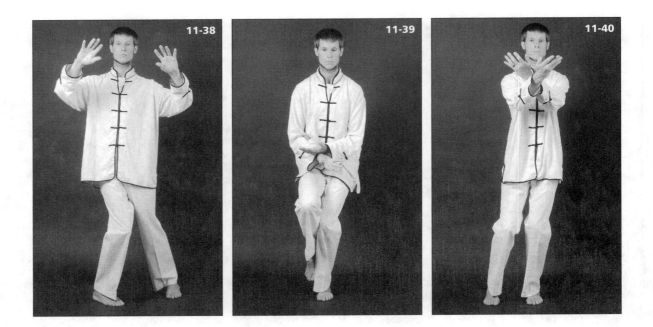

☯ COMPLETE

(Stance type/direction: 50/50 N.) Inhale, separating your arms, palms up, to shoulder width (see **FIGURE 11-41**).

Exhale, rolling your hands over, thumbs up and then inward, and settle your palms to rest on a Pillow of Air in Wu Chi (see **FIGURE 11-42**). Breathe deeply, feeling and relaxing your entire body.

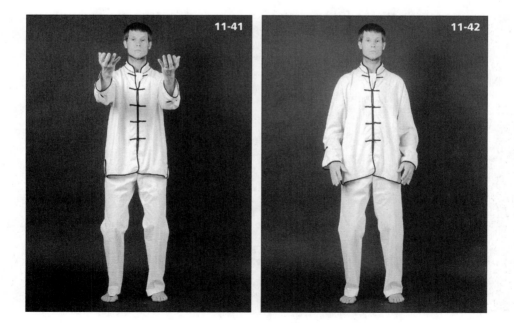

CHAPTER 12
Learning QiGong

QiGong is a very, very old skill, one that has such value that it has been incorporated into virtually every Eastern discipline. Millions of people over the passage of time have enjoyed its gentle benefits. QiGong provides an exceptional advantage to anyone who practices it with diligence and regularity.

Sorting T'ai Chi from QiGong

When T'ai Chi first became popular in the 1960s and 1970s, QiGong was not known. As T'ai Chi was altered to fit this culture's desire for excellent health and reduced stress, the Ch'uan (martial arts portion) was sometimes dropped. This created a T'ai Chi form that was devoted to health, breath, and spiritual awareness. QiGong emerged in the 1990s. QiGong has a form that requires less memorization of different flowing positions than T'ai Chi because QiGong is more stationary.

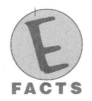

FACTS

Today, a clearly defined line doesn't really exist between T'ai Chi and QiGong. Actually, T'ai Chi (without the Ch'uan) and QiGong carry similarities, and one is not necessarily a precursor to the other as far as which should be learned first. Each is a skill in its own right.

The Importance of Chi

QiGong focuses on drawing in the breath, the carrier of the chi. As chi enters and is dispersed throughout the body, the energy meridians begin to balance through the yin and yang flow, and you feel calmer. The reservoirs for the chi begin to fill, and you feel more alive. The chi is now full enough in your body, and you can begin the chi cultivation process—you feel creative, with plenty of juice.

As you cultivate the chi, the reservoirs of energy stabilize and fill the meridians, and you have more energy to harness and focus. The meridians become plump and rich with chi. Yin and yang flows find their natural balance, given your temperament, and you feel at home with and at peace in yourself. You may find that your weight adjusts to your best body weight for maximum well-being. You may find that time seems more spacious. You may find that simple pleasures in life become more wonderful. You may even find you like—even love—yourself and your life more than ever before. I believe these are the natural birthrights of each one of us.

We have created a culture that doesn't understand or appreciate the lasting benefits of a well-balanced life. There has been, until recently, little support for finding and maintaining one's health using the ancient wisdoms of breath, energy, intent, and self-discipline. QiGong has thrived all these thousands of years because by its very nature it returns us to these basic balances.

Very ancient, early peoples lived on earth when the air was perfect. They lived here when light was not filtered through chemicals. They lived here when exercise was a part of life, when the inner-world connection with one another was stronger and deeper than the outer-world connection. They were closer to the pulses of nature than you can imagine. From this pure environment of breath, light, and chi, QiGong was probably born. They didn't need movement, because that happened all the time. They weren't concerned about the body doing one thing and the mind doing another. Most of the day, the two were working in unison. What has been handed down to us now is a form of reinstating into our bodies the energetic health that's a prerequisite to any fulfilling life, a recipe for a more stable inner life that creates a richer and fuller outer life.

Reviewing the QiGong Exercises

The following QiGong exercises have been put together for you by instructor Fernando Raynolds. He has chosen classic QiGong and a few variations to ensure a complete experience. This selection of QiGong exercises is an excellent introduction to this vast field. It includes meridian stimulation exercises, moving exercises, and stationary stances. Try these exercises in the sequence in which they are presented. After you're able to do an exercise without relying on the book, progress to the next one. The exercises don't need to be done all at the same time, or even in sequence, but they are presented in a sensible sequence here. Running through the sequence in twenty to thirty minutes a day will have a significant impact in your life.

These specific exercises are presented here for a number of reasons:

- Most people experience significant beneficial effects the very first time they do each of these practices.
- Attentive practice can yield profound results.

- These exercises are comparatively easy to learn from a book and don't require a great deal of precision to be beneficial.
- These exercises have no negative side effects.

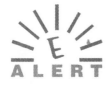

Some people may become a little dizzy or may feel faint from these breathing exercises. If this happens for you, simply sit down and take a rest. If this recurs, check with your doctor.

BREATH STIMULATION

This stimulation is great for asthma or when recovering from cough or cold and increasing respiratory volume. This exercise is performed in order to increase the fullness of the breath (called tidal volume). Most of the time, you breathe unconsciously, and the volume of your breath is determined by the range of motion of your rib cage. This exercise increases your range of motion while also stimulating the air sacs in your lungs. Similar treatments are used therapeutically for respiratory illnesses in both the East and West. This exercise is particularly useful after recovering from a cough, because many people tend to restrict their breathing to prevent coughing. This exercise and the next one make use of a stroke also found in Swedish massage, called tapotment, or tapping yourself.

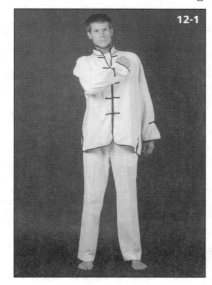

12-1

Take a deep breath in and hold it. Firmly tap yourself either with a fist or open palm all over the surface of the rib cage. (See **FIGURE 12-1**.) Do one side at a time, under your arm, in front of your chest, on your shoulder, and on your back. Then do the other side. As you get comfortable with this exercise, you may find yourself hitting yourself surprisingly firmly, but remember to always be gentle—this shouldn't hurt! Start gently and find the depth that's right for you. And don't hit yourself with your rings or bracelets!

Hold your breath on the inhale for as long as you comfortably can and then release. Do this for a minimum of two breaths. Then rest and feel your body.

MERIDIAN STIMULATION

According to Chinese medicine, there are twelve bilateral meridians and two midline meridians along which the chi, or life energy, flows. Health is determined by the strength and balance of these chi flows. This exercise stimulates the flow of energy on the meridians and is an excellent tonic. It doesn't follow the pathway of the meridians precisely, but is a general treatment of the whole system. It can be used to wake yourself up, because it is quite invigorating.

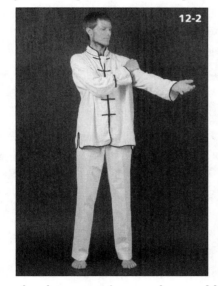
12-2

Again, you are striking yourself, so start gently and find the depth that is right for you. You begin with your arms and slap from your shoulder down the inside of one arm, past the elbow to your wrist and palm (see **FIGURE 12-2**).

Then strike back up from your palm along the outside of your arm, back up to your shoulder. Repeat on your other arm. Strike up the back of the neck and use fingertips on the base of your skull. Using your palms or fingertips, go back and forth over your scalp. Move the face, making sure you get your eyes, cheeks, nose, jaw, and ears. Move on down your neck and throat and thump on your thymus, about a hand's breadth down from the hollow of your throat. Move down your torso to your pelvis, striking down the outsides of your legs, up the insides, down the fronts to the outside of your shin bone, up the insides, down the back of your legs and up the insides. Then beat yourself along the crest of your pelvis to the sides and rear, in the buttocks and in the inguinal area of the groin. There are lots of lymphatic vessels here, so take your time in the inguinal area. From there you slap on your lower back where you can reach and then up and down one side of the body under the armpit. Then finish with the other side.

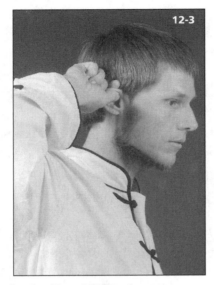
12-3

Having stimulated the whole body, you massage your ears. Put your thumbs in your ears with the index fingers above and squeeze and massage the whole ear (see **FIGURE 12-3**). Make sure to work into all the folds. According to Traditional Chinese Medicine (TCM), there are acupuncture points for the whole body on the ear, so a thorough massage of the ear stimulates the whole body. Finish the ears by brushing them down and back as if pushing the hair behind your ears.

Finish this exercise by stroking your body. You follow the same pattern as the slapping and use a light but satisfying pressure. You begin with your arms and stroke from the shoulder down the inside of one arm, past your elbow to your wrist and palm, then back up from your palm along the outside of your arm and back up to your shoulder. Repeat on the other arm. Stroke up the back of your neck to the base of your skull. Smooth your hair over the scalp. Move down your face, making sure you get your eyes, cheeks, nose, jaw, and ears. Move on down your neck and throat, then down your torso to your pelvis, stroking down the outsides of your legs, up the insides, down the fronts to the outside of your shin bone, up the insides, down the back of your legs, and up the insides. Then move along the crest of the pelvis to the sides and rear, in the buttocks and in the inguinal area of the groin. From there you stroke the lower back where you can reach and then up and down one side of the body under the armpit. Finish with the other side.

After you've completed this exercise, stand for a few moments and simply enjoy the tingling vitality you feel!

HOLDING THE MOON FULL-BODY BREATHING

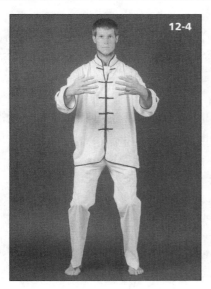

12-4

This exercise mobilizes the chi through the arms, shoulders, and chest while expanding your lungs. This is a mostly stationary exercise, where you stand with your feet parallel, weight evenly distributed, hip- to shoulder-width between the center of your heels. The ankles, knees, and hip joints are positioned so that they are slightly bent and springy, with the knees a little spread so they are over the centerlines of your feet. Your legs are slightly braced so that from the pelvis down, your body feels solid and rooted to the ground. Your arms are *hug* held as if embracing a large beach ball (the moon), with your palms facing *Tree* the chest at out the level of the base of your breast bone. (See **FIGURE 12-4**.)

Once in this posture, breathe deeply and fully, filling your lungs from the base of your abdomen up into your upper chest. Allow your arms to move with the filling and emptying of your lungs. As you inhale, feel and imagine that you're filling your whole body with golden light that energizes a sphere of light surrounded by the arms. The sphere expands on the inhale and contracts on the exhale. As you exhale, feel and imagine your body glowing, radiating that golden light as a blessing out into the universe.

You can do this exercise for up to ten minutes at a time, but start by doing it for ten breaths or so. In any case, stop when your arms grow tired. It is counterproductive to push yourself to endure because it is not a strength-building exercise.

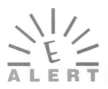

Many people sense warmth, tingling, or magnetism if they hold their hands close to each other after this exercise. Hold your hands as if on either side of a cantaloupe. What do you feel? What happens if you move your hands closer or further apart?

EARTH AND HEAVEN BREATHING

This exercise uses your arms with your breathing as in Holding the Moon Full-Body Breathing, but here you go up and down with your breath. The movements should be smooth and your arms as relaxed and open as possible.

You start with the Earth portion of this exercise. According to Traditional Chinese Medicine, the Yin energy of the Earth doesn't have a particular emotional tone to it—it is simply vital energy—while the yang energy from the heavens has more of a positive emotional charge to it. For this reason, you start with Earth breathing and then bring in the inspiration of the heavens.

Standing in the same posture for the legs as described in Holding the Moon Full-Body Breathing, use your arms to draw energy up from the Earth on the inhale and radiate it out on the exhale. Your hands are drawn up the midline, fingers touching, palms up, a few inches from your body. (See **FIGURE 12-5**.)

At about mid-chest, your palms must turn, going from facing up, to facing the body, to facing down, to facing away, to facing up again. Your hands go up above your head as far as is comfortable (see **FIGURE 12-6**) and then separate on the exhale, slowly dropping, palms down, to the

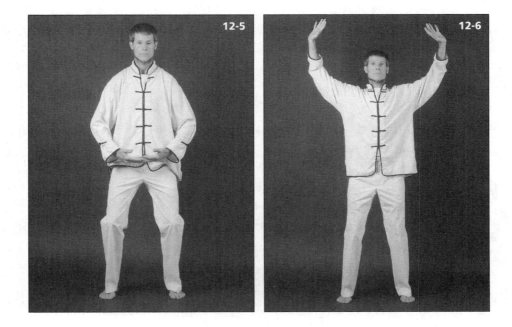

sides. Allow your whole body to compress down, bending your knees more at the end of the exhale to reach a little lower and gather the Earth energy. And as your hands go up, allow the legs to straighten. You feel and image drawing the Earth energy up through the body, and as you exhale, you imagine it fountaining out the crown of the head from your entire body.

Do this for three to ten breaths and then change the direction of the circles drawn by the arms to do the Heaven portion of this exercise. Standing in the same posture for the legs, gather energy in from the universe and push it down through the body, through the soles of the feet into the earth. Your arms go up at the sides on the inhale, palms forward. (See **FIGURE 12-7**.)

Your arms then go to vertical and, when exhaling, come down the right and left sides of the body with about an inch and a half between the fingertips (see **FIGURE 12-8**). Again, on the exhale, your hands travel within an inch or so of the front of your body. Feel and imagine gathering a radiant sphere of universal energy into the arms on your inhale, and then draw and push the energy down through the right and left sides and from there into the center of the Earth. Allow your legs to straighten a bit as your arms go up and deepen the bend at your knees as your arms go down.

Do the Heaven part of this cycle for three to ten breaths and then stand quietly for a moment to savor the effect.

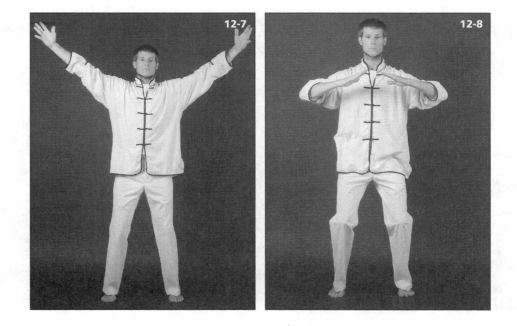

SWIMMING DRAGON

This is a more complicated exercise that balances the energy, exercises the spine, and trains balance and breath control. T. K. Shih, who has written a book on this practice, also cites it as a weight-control exercise. Stand with your feet parallel and together, knees slightly bent.

Bring the hands together in prayer (with a little pressure between them) below the crotch, fingers pointing down (see **FIGURE 12-9**), and bring them up the centerline, brushing up your body. At about the solar plexus (the area of the abdomen just below the sternum) your hands have to turn, going from fingers down to fingers pointing away from the body to fingers up.

Bring your hands up your left cheek, and then a little forward as they continue to rise to the peak of your reach. Counterbalance this forward reach with your arms with a slight sit in your pelvis. (See **FIGURE 12-10**.)

Then your hands come down your right cheek and cross horizontally at your neck, moving to the left. Keep your right forearm horizontal and your wrist straight, and counterbalance this movement by moving your hips right and looking right. (See **FIGURE 12-11**.)

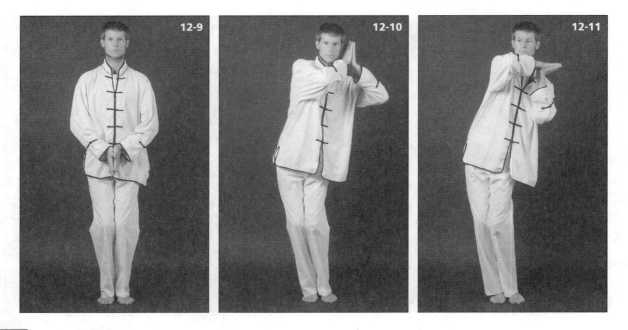

12-9

12-10

12-11

Lower your hands, fingertips down, and cross at the solar plexus going right. Counterbalance this movement by swinging your hips left and looking left. (See **FIGURE 12-12**.)

Again, lower your hands and cross now at the groin (see **FIGURE 12-13**), with your eyes and hips counterbalancing by swinging right (see **FIGURE 12-14**).

Raise your hands a bit to cross again at the solar plexus, with your eyes and hips swinging left.

Cross your hands again at the throat, right forearm horizontal, with your gaze and hips swinging right to counterbalance (see **FIGURE 12-15**). Once past your throat, your hands go back up your left cheek and straight overhead. Extend from the flat of your feet to the tips of your fingertips. (See **FIGURE 12-16**.)

Push through the balls of your feet to stand on your toes, stretching from toes to fingertips. Now release and bring your hands down the midline, ending up with your palms flat on your abdomen, your thumbs touching a little below your navel. (See **FIGURE 12-17**.) Rest here for a few breaths.

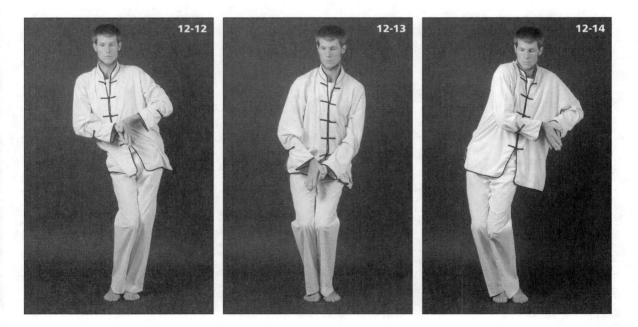

Work on making the movement smooth and flowing like a swimming dragon. As your hands go up, inhale. As your hands go down, exhale and bend your knees while keeping your spine as vertical as the counterbalancing allows. Don't bend over. As your hands switch to going up again, inhale slowly in order to be able to inhale through to the stretch from toes to fingertips. Exhale and breathe freely as your hands settle to your abdomen. As your hands rest on the abdomen, feel and visualize an exchange of loving-kindness energy from the center of both palms into the center of your body.

When I first learned this exercise, I was startled at how centering and calming it was for me. You should be able to notice this effect in three to seven repetitions. Shih recommends an hour a day, one minute per repetition, for weight loss.

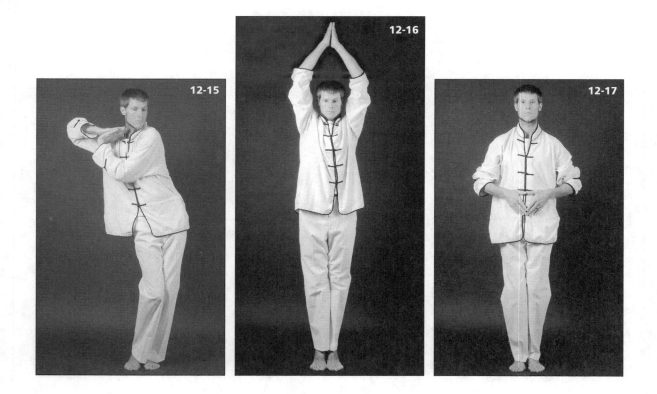

SPAGHETTI ARMS WITH WEIGHT SHIFT

This is an excellent exercise for building a solid stance and also helps you loosen your shoulders and arms while massaging the internal organs of your abdomen. This exercise also makes you more aware of the momentum involved in your body movements. You start this exercise by standing with one foot forward, one foot back, turned slightly out. This stance is also described in Chapter 10 in the 70/30 stance and the 100 Percent Back stance. With your weight mostly forward, your rear heel should be hip- to shoulder-width to the side, as well as comfortably behind. Your ankle, knee, and hip joints should be slightly flexed and springy, and your crotch should be slightly rounded to bring your knees over your feet and create a slight sense of being braced. You then shift your weight back and forth and allow your arms to swing relaxed from your shoulders. As you shift your weight forward, your arms go across your forward leg. (See **FIGURE 12-18**.)

As you shift your weight back, your arms go across your rear leg. (See **FIGURE 12-19**.)

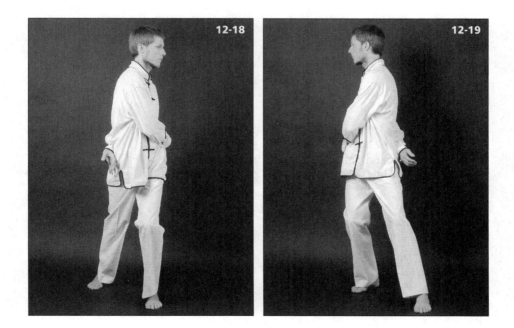

Don't allow your twisting momentum to twist your weighted leg or it will undermine your balance. **FIGURE 12-20** shows the front knee twisted and the rear knee collapsed in. **FIGURE 12-21** shows the rear knee twisted and the front knee collapsed. Be very careful not to do this as it can damage your knees.

Do this exercise for a few minutes on each side, breathing comfortably and relaxing your arms. There are other variations of this exercise: one done in the same stance but twisting the waist so that your arms go the opposite way, over the unweighted leg; another done with your feet parallel and shoulder width apart instead of with one foot forward. After you understand the dynamics of this first one, allow yourself to experiment with the variations. Just be attentive to the safety of your knees!

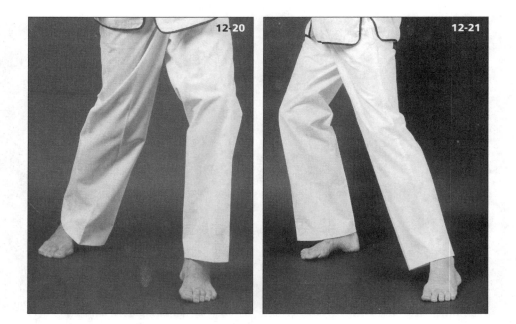

☯ ARM SWINGING UP AND DOWN

Whereas the preceding exercise worked with the momentum of your arms twisting around your spine, this one works with their momentum going up and down. This exercise is good for relaxing your arms, and will also tone your muscles and vitalize your energy along the spine.

You start with your feet parallel, hip- to shoulder-width apart, with your arms at your side. First bend and then straighten your legs, step forward, and transfer that momentum to your free-swinging arms. Begin by stretching your arms up in front of your body. (See **FIGURE 12-22**.) You then drop your arms while you bend your knees (see **FIGURE 12-23**) and straighten your legs and send your arms swinging behind you (see **FIGURE 12-24**).

Again, drop your arms, bend your knees, straighten your legs, and send your arms swinging in front again. As your arms reach the top of their swing to either the front or the back, your legs are

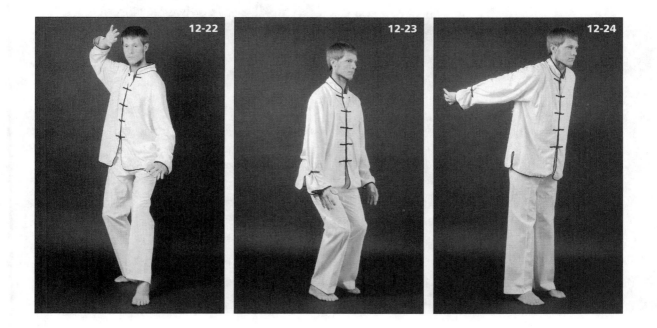

12-22   12-23   12-24

straightened; as your arms are down in line with your body, your knees are bent. Inhale with your arms stretched above in front and exhale as you start the downward arc. Start the next inhale with the downward arc of your arms from the rear. Do this movement at a comfortable pace that doesn't interfere with the momentum. Start the exercise keeping the spine vertical, but after you're comfortable with it, you can begin bending at the waist as your hands go back behind you (see **FIGURE 12-25**) and arching the back as the hands come up in front (see **FIGURE 12-26**).

Do this exercise for about ten repetitions at first, and progress to as many as forty. Make sure you breathe comfortably and that you maintain your sense of connection with the earth through your feet. After you've completed your set, stand quietly and allow your breath and heart rate to settle as you feel your entire body.

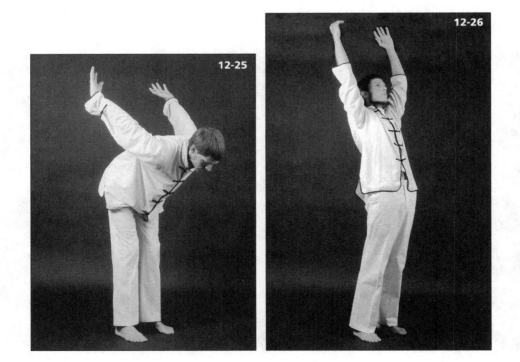

12-25

12-26

☯ CLEANSING WALK

This exercise helps open your breath, build balance, and harmonize the energy down the right and left sides of your body. You start in a stance with your weight in your right leg, with your foot turned out slightly. Your left foot has no weight in it and rests on the ball comfortably in front. On the inhale, you swing your arms up, gathering energy (see **FIGURE 12-27**). On the exhale, you bring your arms down, palms down, along the front of the left side (see **FIGURE 12-28**).

You feel and visualize that you're settling the energy you gathered through the left side and out through the ball of your foot. By running this energy through, you clean out any blocked or grubby energy. Turning your right foot slightly out, you shift your weight into the left foot and swing your right leg forward to rest on the ball. Use the momentum of the weight shift to initiate the upward-gathering movement of your arms. Inhale vitalizing energy and as you exhale, settle that energy down and out through the ball of your right foot. Feel and visualize the energy moving through and cleansing the internal organs on each side of the body.

Do this seven to twenty times on each side. Then come to rest and feel your body.

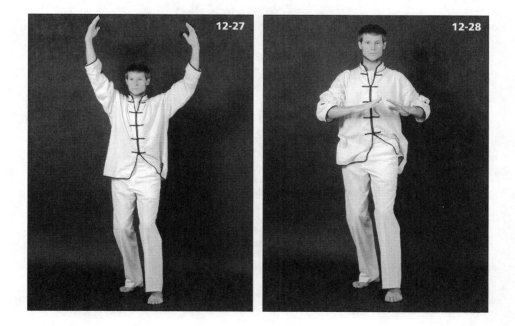

12-27   12-28

☯ WU CHI

The name Wu Chi refers to the formlessness that precedes the separation of the primal energies into the fundamental duality of yin and yang. As you stand in this meditation (see **FIGURE 12-29**), you are seeking to return to a sense of formlessness by allowing the boundaries of your body and ego to dissolve. This is one of the best exercises for truly understanding how to relax on all levels as well as teaching profound truths about your relationship with gravity and the proper use of the will.

The postural requirements are as follows: feet parallel, hip- to shoulder-width apart; ankles, knees, and hips bent and loose, sinking from the tan t'ien (see Chapter 1); and pelvis down through the soles of your feet. Your weight is evenly distributed on your feet, right to left, heel to toe, and side to side. Then lightly extend your spine through the crown of your head, shoulders resting on your rib cage and the rib cage mobile with your breath. Your tongue lightly touches the roof of your mouth and allows your neck to be free, your head floats with your chin slightly tucked. You may choose to have your eyes gently open or lightly

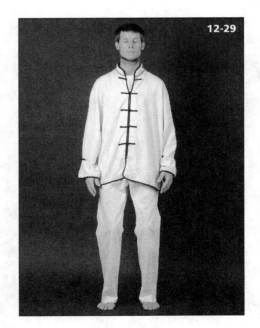

12-29

closed. After you're in Wu Chi, bring looseness to your joints by breathing deeply and bringing the movement of the breath into your whole body. From the outside, you should appear to be standing still, but from the inside, you should feel your whole body mobile with the breath.

ESSENTIALS

It takes most people a while to become comfortable in Wu Chi. Most of us have habitual tension patterns that show up as pain and blocked energy when we simply stand still. Working with this exercise will help you understand and release these areas, but patience and compassion with yourself is required.

Slowly allow your mind to rest on the vertical line of extension through the core of your body and refer all sensations to that line and down into the earth. As with any meditation process, if your mind drifts away, simply bring it back to focus without judgment or surprise.

Stand for as long as you're comfortable—this is not an endurance test. The next time you stand, see if you can incorporate what you learned from the previous time and stand for a little longer. Those who really pursue Wu Chi as a core practice often stand for up to an hour a day.

ROCKING ON THE BALLS OF THE FEET

This is a powerful exercise for tuning into your balance and feeling and allowing the natural flow of movement in your body. For some, it can bring up some anxiety about control, so be especially gentle with yourself. You set this exercise up by putting your body in Wu Chi (see the preceding section), and then shifting most of your weight to the balls of your feet. As you breathe and relax your entire body, the body will start to swaying with the breath. For most people, this starts right away, but don't be concerned if it takes a few breaths. As the body starts to sway, simply allow it to do so. Keep breathing and relaxing and work to completely release control over the sway while maintaining the structure of your posture.

ALERT

Do this exercise only after you understand the basics of Wu Chi, and then start with just a few minutes of practice. There is no great benefit to doing this exercise for more than seven minutes.

This exercise can serve as a stepping-off point for the practice of spontaneous QiGong, which is an approach where you feel and follow the natural flow of your energy into whatever kind of movement feels right. In order to explore this more, take either the Earth and Heaven Breathing or the Holding the Moon posture and allow these exercises to be the themes upon which you, like a jazz musician, improvise. If this is enjoyable and comfortable for you, allow yourself to also explore vocalizing with the movement. Adding this element can be more emotionally evocative. Doing this kind of spontaneous QiGong is inappropriate if you have unresolved emotional illness or trauma.

CHAPTER 13

Push-Hands—
Look into My Eyes

This chapter is devoted to a unique aspect of T'ai Chi, the Push-Hands. In most partnership exercises the focus is to overwhelm the other person and win. In Push-Hands, the focus is to understand your partner nonverbally, and take that understanding into achieving greater empathy. Push-Hands provides a safe world in which new styles of responding to life and other people can be experimented with.

Understanding Push-Hands

Push-Hands is the name most often used to describe a variety of two-person exercises used in T'ai Chi. Often each person is trying to cause the other to lose balance while following a more or less complicated series of movements. Although Push-Hands practice has lost most of its martial arts applications, it is an important aspect of training because it is in the confrontation with another that your skills are really tested. Just how good is your balance? Just how sensitive and relaxed are you? In addition, it can be delightful to play Push-Hands with a well-matched partner.

ESSENTIAL

Each person will become themselves in their own individual style of Push-Hands: Some push; others won't push at all. Some move before they are pushed; still others won't be pushed at all. All these are personal styles of being in the world.

Many emotional issues may arise as you practice Push-Hands. After all, your partner may be trying to push you over. It is easy to get ticked off and uptight if you are consistently "losing," or you may just not be comfortable having another person in your space. It is not unusual to be confronted with your own fear, anger, or self-judgment when practicing Push-Hands. Because of this, it is important to choose a partner with whom you feel comfortable. Consider how aggressive, competitive, and sensitive your partner is. If you can find a partner with whom you feel emotionally safe, you will feel comfortable sharing and exploring more personal aspects of your training and it will be a far richer experience for you.

Much of the T'ai Chi training curriculum is based on slowly increasing the level of stress within which you can relax. As you learn to relax in the simpler Push-Hands drills, you can move on to more complex ones.

A L E R T

Always push slowly and gently and do not poke. The pusher should work on his or her sensitivity to pushing as the person being pushed works on his sensitivity to being pushed. As you become familiar with yielding to the push by shifting back and turning, invite your partner to push closer to your centerline.

Doing Push-Hands Drills

As with the rest of T'ai Chi, different styles and teachers have their own Push-Hands drills. This section gives you a sampling of how this part of T'ai Chi works.

The following drills are meant to be done slowly and with sensitivity. For the most part, the slower you go, the more you will learn, but also let yourself practice moving more quickly. In general, the amount of pressure in a push is determined by the person who is yielding, so if you're pushing, push gently and allow the pressure to build up to the level your partner chooses. If you're being pushed, determine the strength of the push by how quickly you yield to it. If you don't move out of the way, the pressure should build.

Special thanks to student Ann Ramage for posing with Fernando on these Push-Hands drills.

There are a variety of warm-up drills for Push-Hands. For the most part, they involve feeling a slow linear push and moving to yield to it while keeping the stance solid. Generally the person receiving the push starts in a 70/30 posture. The pusher may stand in a similar posture

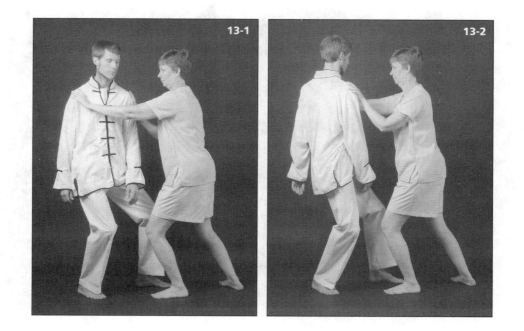

within easy reach, or he may be free to move around (see **FIGURES 13-1** and **13-2**). Pushes are easier to yield to the further out from the center line they are, so it is best to start pushing on shoulders or hips and move closer to the center as your partner becomes more experienced. The person being pushed can also cross his or her arms across the chest or put hands on the shoulders to provide a surface on which to be pushed.

After you're comfortable with this first drill, add another level of complexity by eliminating the requirement that the push be linear. Now your partner is free to change the direction of the push as you yield to it. This drill is called Seeking Center. It's a little like trying to keep an inflated ball underwater—as you push the ball down it will roll and spin to come up—to keep it under, you'll need to compensate. Similarly, as you are pushed and yield, your partner compensates in order to keep pushing you over. This drill is best done slowly. After one person is knocked over, switch roles (see **FIGURES 13-3** and **13-4**).

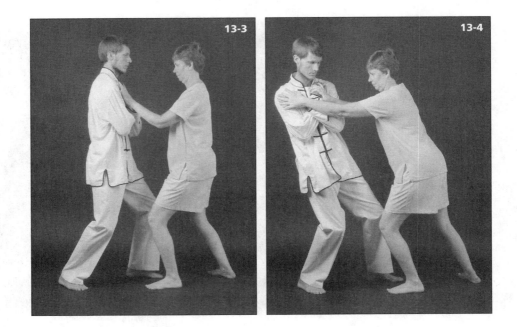

☯ BASIC ONE-HANDED WATER DRILL

For the most part, physical attacks are linear like the flight of an arrow, as opposed to the preceding drill, which is like the flight of an attacking bee. In this drill, you mimic yielding to a punch, which is a linear attack. Both people stand in a 70/30 posture within easy reach. Both people have the right foot forward and the right hand forward touching at the wrist. (See **FIGURE 13-5**.)

As one person moves to push, his hand turns to face his partner. Her palm turns to face herself in a Ward Off. (See **FIGURE 13-6**.)

The person who is being pushed shifts into his rear leg and deflects the incoming push to the side. (See **FIGURE 13-7**.)

The roles then reverse, and he comes forward to push her. The pusher concentrates on delivering a linear push to where his partner's centerline was when he initiated the push. If seen from above, the point of contact at the wrists should move back and forth essentially on a line. When your legs or arms tire, switch sides. An important aspect of this drill is to maintain feet, leg, and pelvis alignment throughout. It is very easy to get distracted and end up twisting your knees.

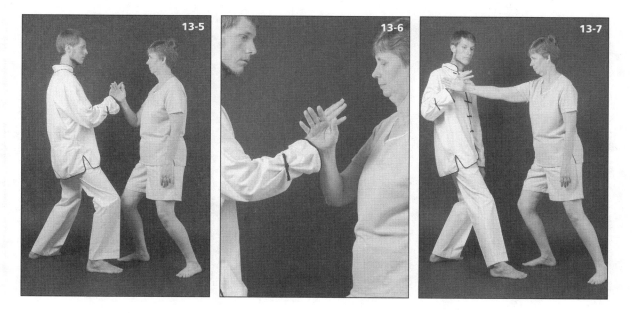

ONE-STEP WATER DRILL

This drill makes the practice a little more intense by allowing the pusher to take one step forward and the person being pushed one step back. This mimics an attacker stepping in and punching with the forward hand. Both people are again in a 70/30 facing each other, but this time they are mirrors of each other—one with the left foot forward, one with the right. Both use either the right or left arms and the hands again touch at the wrist. (See **FIGURE 13-8**.)

Using the right arms, the person with the left foot forward steps forward with the right foot pushing linearly to the partner's centerline. The partner steps back and deflects (see **FIGURE 13-9**).

Now the roles reverse. (See **FIGURE 13-10**.) Repeat, starting nice and slowly, and if you like, building up speed and intensity.

Keep the pressure between the hands light by yielding. Keep the attack linear. Continue to pay attention to the solidity of your stance and maintain feet, leg, and pelvis alignment as you step back and forth. When you tire, use the other arm. For the left arm, the person with the right foot forward will step and push first.

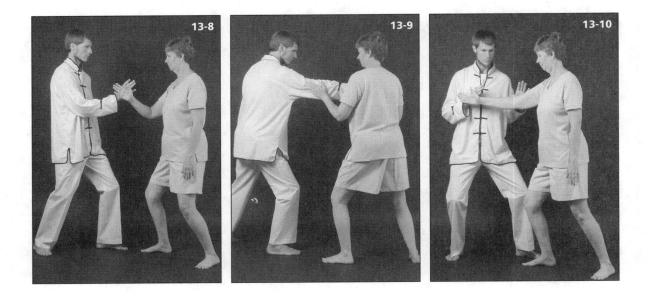

13-8   13-9   13-10

ROLL BACK

Another step in practicing T'ai Chi with another person is to take one or more movements and practice them on each other. These kinds of exercises range from single movement drills all the way to quite complex two person forms. This one described here is a drill for the downward drag of Roll Back.

In this drill, the people stand 90 degrees apart from each other. The person on the right drags the other's right arm by holding the wrist with her right hand and the elbow with her left. By levering down, she pulls him toward the floor. (See **FIGURE 13-11**.)

He steps in with his right to catch himself and then brings the left leg in to improve his support. At the same time, he drops his right elbow and raises the hand to disrupt her grasp. (See **FIGURE 13-12**.)

Twisting his right hand to grab her wrist, he steps around behind himself with his right foot, pushing back with the left leg and using that power to drag her arm, positioning his left hand on her elbow. He is now 90 degrees in front of her, pulling her into the dirt (see **FIGURE 13-13**). She steps in with her right foot to catch herself, and the cycle continues.

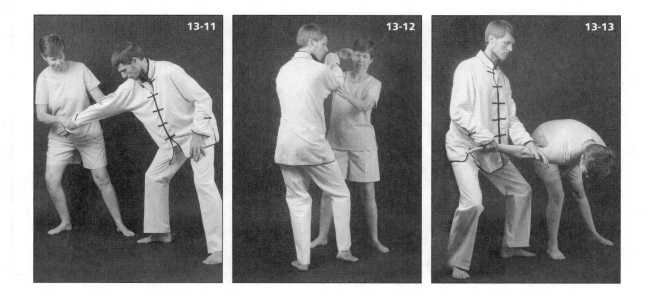

13-11 13-12 13-13

After you've practiced the movements, Push-Hands can be done quite quickly and strongly, but start out slowly and gently. Stay mindful of your stance, and keep your body upright.

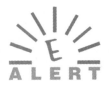

Many aspects of Push-Hands can be learned from a book or video. However, the need for a watchful instructor is absolutely critical with Push-Hands. Use this book to become familiar with some of the positions, movements, and concepts of push and receive, but seek out a live instructor before going much deeper.

CHAPTER 14

Combining T'ai Chi with Sex and Pregnancy

Sharing the movement of T'ai Chi between partners can intensely improve a couple's sex life. Because of the emphasis on self-discipline, there are guidelines about how to arrive at these peak moments of bliss and ecstasy. T'ai Chi is also a wonderful exercise to sustain an enjoyable pregnancy and facilitate a more comfortable birth.

Understanding Chi

Chi is the force of life. Besides air, there are other sources from which we draw chi. Chi is in the food we eat and the liquids we drink. We draw it up and absorb it from the earth and draw it down and into our bodies from the universe. T'ai Chi and QiGong were skillfully designed to increase one's ability to cultivate chi and then heighten the qualities of chi within.

Chi comes in many forms. Low vibrating chi carries undesirable emotions like rage and possessiveness. Low vibrating chi binds one to a life of reduced spiritual value. High vibrating chi carries within it the ability to have a perspective on life and one's place in it that makes lower form emotions as outdated as lumbering, extinct dinosaurs. The martial arts schools all had masters who had attained this level of consciousness through self-mastery and T'ai Chi Ch'uan mastery. Seeing, learning from, and understanding what mastery looks and feels like was a big motivator to the others in the school.

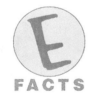

FACTS

Each aspect of life came under the scrutiny of self-discipline. The martial arts, eating, communication, the arts, gardening, and even sex were all embraced as opportunities to further one's self-mastery and heighten chi within and have perfect discipline in the outer world. Heightening one's self-awareness to engage chi was the core of the experience.

In addition to drawing in personal chi, we also gain chi from co-mingling with another person's chi. This occurs in any contact in which the boundaries of the self are softened or lowered. They are times when a relationship with another melts or destroys the boundaries around the self. Hugging, laughing together, sharing the pleasure of eating, holding hands, carrying a child, working as or with an energy healer are some ways in which the boundaries soften or melt.

Physical abuse also creates co-mingling and will destroy boundaries. Abuse is the result of the abuser engaging low vibrating chi. To suffer from abuse can cause long-term problems with clear self-knowledge. This provides a great reason to come into an understanding of chi. Through

T'ai Chi and QiGong, the lower chi absorbed when the abuse occurred can be elevated, and inner freedom from the abuse can be attained.

ESSENTIALS

The co-mingling that produces the highest form of chi is characterized by a sweet pleasure and relaxed feeling of harmony, union, and knowing one's place in the scheme of things. Sex was considered to offer the most heightened state of co-mingling chi.

When two people talk, chi begins to pass back and forth between them. If this conversation is heightened by a mutual physical attraction, the chi begins to circulate between them faster. If the attraction increases to arousal, the chi has increased in momentum. This creates an intense and usually compelling magnetic flow of energy between the two people.

Improving the Sexual Union

T'ai Chi Ch'uan students were taught that there was an enhanced way to approach sexual union. This approach would ensure that the sexual experience would be life-enhancing and spiritually sustaining for both partners.

Mastery of one's self was the path to spiritual enlightenment. The goal of the martial artist is useful here to understand the goal for sexual union. The ideal was to be so skillful that in the height of battle, the heat and passion of the fighting never swept the warrior into emotionally driven action. The warrior was centered himself in his self-awareness, exhibited through his disciplined skill and heightened chi as he used the emotionally charged environment to center into inner stillness ever more deeply. The more emotional the scene became, the calmer he got. The bottom line is that all of life is a journey for us to continually cultivate and heighten chi. Each experience life gives us is another golden opportunity to elevate our qualities as people. This path could conceivably become pretty self-absorbed were it not for sex!

This co-mingling of chi the T'ai Chi Ch'uan masters taught was the gift of perfect autonomy in perfect union with others. This was seen as the most exalted of unions. It was also seen as a very critical union in intent, process, and outcome. Calmness, control, and mastery over the self, in both partners, was the key to higher states of experience.

ALERT

If sexuality is expressed incorrectly, one or both parties is drained of the vital and health-generating chi. When the sexuality is driven by little mastery over the body and high desire, it produces anxiety and frustration. A few ways this can show up is as possessiveness, jealousy, selfishness, and controlling behavior.

T'ai Chi Ch'uan teachers believed that chi was in a very concentrated form in the egg/yin and the sperm/yang. As the sexual chi between the partners increases in momentum, the partners come closer and closer to orgasm. This concentrated chi in the egg and sperm join into this energetic dance of life and regeneration. The moment of orgasm is the culmination of this momentum. To be unable to reach this peak was seen as a problem with tension or energy imbalance.

The prescribed guidelines and ensuing discipline were derived from a close examination of this chi dance to orgasm. Because the egg is internal within the woman, she was encouraged to have an orgasm. It was felt the internal state of the egg combined with the internal beginnings of the orgasm enhanced the egg and gave the woman more rejuvenating chi for her own spiritual benefit. This chi co-mingled with her partner's chi.

Males were encouraged to orgasm with ejaculation only when wanting to produce a child. The ejaculation of the sperm out of the man and into the woman created a loss of chi for the man. This loss of chi was taken very seriously, and men were taught to develop sexual mastery to curtail this loss. They were taught how to engage in longer and longer sexual unions. By achieving a calm mind and a relaxed inner state, these times of longer sexual union did not culminate in ejaculation. Instead, a heightened sense of sexual refinement and spiritual pleasure was achieved. This then became a different type of orgasm, free of tension-relieving ejaculation, now with a new spiritual significance. The chi would then heighten to a point where bliss was experienced throughout the sexual union.

This delay of the rush to orgasm placed a heightened emphasis on the role of eroticism. Eroticism evolved as an art form in itself. Eroticism led to arousal. Arousal became heightened through prolonged touching. As the chi intensified its momentum, the T'ai Chi was there. Yin and yang separated, and true union was at hand. Each partner emerged filled with better health, longevity, and access to a state of bliss, a bliss that can only be experienced (no words do it justice). When this marvelous union was attained, each person became and shared the embodiment of T'ai Chi and separating yin and yang.

E

FACTS

Taoists studied everything thoroughly and drew all of life into a circle of life in which all affected everything and nothing was separate and isolated. Sexual arts became a part of this circle.

Different sexual positions were prescribed to enhance the health and well-being of different organs. Breathing was seen in two parts—getting the breath in the lungs and then permeating the entire body with chi—as was sex. First the arousal, then specific positions were taken to encourage the chi to drive more deeply into a depleted organ.

Shallow and casual sex were not helpful in increasing personal mastery and heightened awareness. Sex where arousal and desire were driven by substances was seen as fraught with peril because of the dangerously low vibrating chi associated with it.

The ideal was to have both partners committed to their own development, committed to finding bliss through union with each other, and then committed to refining over time this discipline of sex. With the partners relaxed and mutually sustaining, an environment of spiritual development emerged in an atmosphere of blissful union.

Practicing T'ai Chi and QiGong During Pregnancy

Pregnancy is such an important time for having balance and harmony within. The fetus is affected by each event that occurs to the parents, in particular the mother. If the mother has an upsetting experience but her body is well balanced, filled with chi, and in accord with the yin and yang flows, she still provides a protected and positive environment for her unborn child. It is a safe harbor amidst the constant changes of life.

This is similar to a home providing a welcome refuge, a safe harbor amidst the constant changes of life. A peaceful home that provides a welcome refuge can be a home that has been shaped by the Chinese art of placement, Feng Shui (see Chapter 20). This ancient wisdom enlists the ancient Chinese understanding of elements, chi, and harmony in household decorating. A home that has followed the rules of Feng Shui has a quality of peace and harmony that other homes do not have. This is a perfect metaphor for an expectant mother who adds T'ai Chi into her prenatal program. Establish in the body an inner environment of balance, harmony, and increased chi, and you will enhance your pregnancy. You will also improve the inner environment for your baby.

As for birth, it can be rigorous, and having your breath open and relaxed, your chi fuller, and a previously established, safe environment for you and your baby will make it an easier process.

FACTS

You do not need any special instruction to practice during your pregnancy. The normal T'ai Chi movements and the QiGong breathing are perfect. As your belly gets bigger you will have to accommodate somewhat, but not enough to diminish the positive gifts of T'ai Chi and QiGong.

If you live near a T'ai Chi teacher, you may be able to find a class held just for pregnant women. It is really fun to do T'ai Chi and QiGong with others having the same experience. You can follow any exercise in the book. Be especially careful you've provided a safe area of movement for yourself so you absolutely can't fall over or down. Make a safe, well lit, and spacious environment in which to learn, relax, and enjoy.

And congratulations!

CHAPTER 15
Kids Can Do It, Too

In China, children learn T'ai Chi and QiGong by watching older people as they practice. T'ai Chi has become so popular in China anyone can see it done from morning to evening in any park. T'ai Chi can be fun for children and provide them with many of the benefits adults receive.

Including Your Kids in T'ai Chi

The value of T'ai Chi is the same for children as for anyone (see Chapter 3), but it is a rare child who will want to learn the traditional form. T'ai Chi was never adapted to children in the traditional form. Now, however, it is adapted in a way that children can learn to improve their balance, increase their coordination, improve interaction skills, and discover energetic sensitivity. For naturally energetically sensitive children it can be very worthwhile to have those gentle but powerful sensitivities validated and learn to utilize them.

FACTS

In a culture devoted to the fine arts and martial arts, T'ai Chi Ch'uan in ancient China was a secret, revered training. The natural tendency to hero worship was directed toward the men who advanced in these arts. As T'ai Chi became more attainable to everyone in the 1900s, children would see single men "dancing" with the wind and from a distance, would try to emulate them.

Focusing on Fun

It is rare for children younger than sixteen to really enjoy the careful process of learning and practicing T'ai Chi. Although some younger kids will be attracted to learning the form, for the most part, children enjoy the simpler exercises, including the warm-ups, stretches, and QiGong, as well as the two-person drills from T'ai Chi.

As is true for adults, for children to practice attentively, the practice must be enjoyable as well as meaningful. Many of the practices can be tailored more for kids simply by using a more playful attitude and creating games from the movements. Most children have rich imaginations, and their imagery and visualization can make the movements more fun.

Improving Balance

As a parent or teacher, your goal for your child may be to help her improve balance, coordination, and self confidence while developing a feel for her own energy. Many children will also experience an increased ability to slow down and concentrate. But the children themselves, for the most part, will be more motivated by social concerns and simply having fun.

Doing Warm-Ups

With a little creativity and enthusiasm from a leader, kids enjoy doing warm-ups. For example, with the wrist and ankle swirls, kids can try to unscrew their hands and feet. (In addition, because children tend to be looser and more flexible than adults, these exercises can be done faster and with fewer repetitions than described in other chapters.) Imaginative and humorous presentations will help children engage with QiGong exercises, as well. The breath stimulation, for example, can be presented as Tarzan training.

It can also be helpful to take a leisurely pace with children and start the movements out being quite free and unspecified and only later start teaching a more specific series. For example, Swimming Dragon can begin with movements where the arms are brought together as a single snake, and then the whole body simply gets snaky (see **FIGURE 15-1**).

Spaghetti arm swings can develop from playing with the pacing, lumbering movements of an upright bear (see **FIGURE 15-2**).

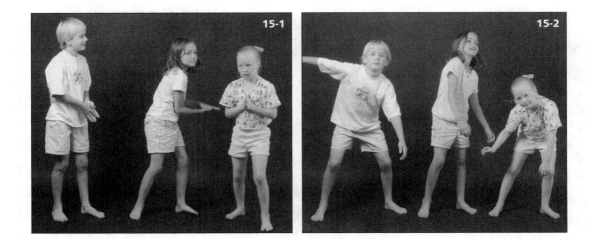

Wu Chi can develop in imaginative exercises of rooting like a tree and rocking on the balls of the feet from visualizing the body as seaweed or a candle flame (see **FIGURE 15-3**).

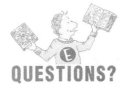

QUESTIONS?

How can I get my child to practice T'ai Chi?
Children are often uninterested in practicing the movements. In addition to keeping the practice fun, consider opening your child's practice to a larger group of people, even of widely varied age ranges.

Children can be very sensitive, and many need only a little encouragement to feel and explore their chi. The breathing with visualization QiGong exercises, such as Holding the Moon and Earth and Heavens, can be powerful doorways for them. After playing with the exercises, kids can be encouraged to visualize and feel a softball-sized sphere of energy between their palms (see **FIGURE 15-4**).

After they have found it, this ball can be stretched and compressed and moved about—even tossed from hand to hand or person to person (see **FIGURE 15-5**).

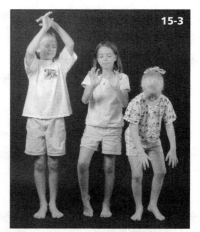

15-3

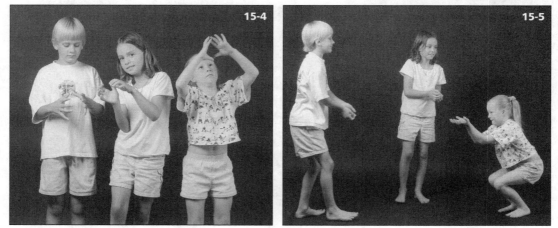

15-4

15-5

Using an Imaginative Presentation

For many children, especially younger ones, T'ai Chi basics are a little dry to hold their attention. Still, imaginative presentation such as using the metaphor of being on a ship on a rolling sea for the solid stance can make this more palatable. Many children will enjoy playing with the balance skills needed to keep the weight 100 percent in one foot or to reach a leg out with no weight. Variations on "red light, green light," where the child must freeze on "red light," can make this more fun.

With a little bit of creativity, "follow the leader" can also be used to make the material more engaging. This may include standing in a circle and having the leader swing her arms in a way that uses her momentum or engages the whole body, having the leader do balance drills of her choice, or using the game to work with the more specified movements of the form.

Playing Games

Two of the fundamental skills developed in T'ai Chi Push-Hands are sensing the other person's movement and allowing your own body to move with it while not sacrificing your structure. These skills lend themselves very nicely to games.

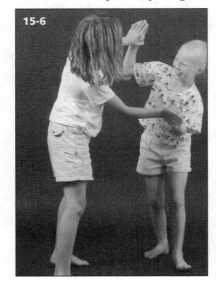

15-6

One example is Palm Dancing, where people stand facing each other with palms against each other. Maintaining gentle contact between the palms, one person moves his hands and the other person follows (see **FIGURE 15-6**). After a few minutes of this, the roles are reversed.

If you want to expand on this idea, have each person lead with the right hand and follow with the left. Again after a few minutes, the roles can be reversed. When only one person is leading, allow that person to move her feet and require her partner to follow.

A variation on this activity is called Glued Together: Two people stick together at any point, and then one moves around while the other follows. The elbows are a good starting point (see **FIGURE 15-7**), but you can try gluing one child's ear to another's shoulder or any of a myriad of options. Chains of children can be made this way too, much to everyone's delight. You can combine a balance game with a trust circle by having two children in the middle surrounded by a circle of children. One of the two in the middle stands while the other tries to lightly push her over into the supporting hands of the other kids. This game can really help a child let her body go. This can be done in a smaller circle as well, where one child is in the middle and gets gently pushed across the circle (see **FIGURE 15-8**). If the child in the middle is comfortable enough, she can even close her eyes to amplify the trust required to really let go.

As kids work with Push-Hands exercises, it is very important that the exercises be designed to minimize competition and to maximize the sense of cooperation, play, and shared discovery. This is ideally what happens in Push-Hands partnerships for adults, as well (see Chapter 13).

Your children may ask questions after you've taught them fun adaptation of T'ai Chi, but more likely, they will want to take what they have learned and apply it. This is good. Walking on the tops of short walls may become very interesting. Coordination games—pat the head/circle the tummy—may come more to the fore. This will be using

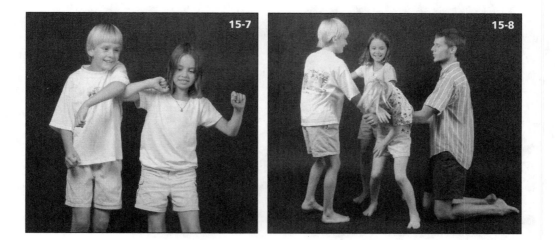

15-7   15-8

their T'ai Chi to integrate a finer motor development into their life for their own pleasure.

In addition, social interactions may bring up questions or complaints about their peers. This provides a good time to learn more about your child's strengths and weaknesses. You can take this opportunity to give them ongoing skills and encouragement as they come to terms with the great complexities of society.

Helping Energetically Sensitive Kids

For energetically sensitive kids, T'ai Chi experiences can be a great help. If a child is energetically sensitive, he or she may have feelings about another person that aren't easily understood but should be validated as worthy. When your child says, "I don't like Janie," you can say, "Why?" He may say, after a thoughtful pause, "I don't know—I just don't." His energetically sensitive feelings may have told him that behind Janie's smile is a mean streak or that Janie has a neediness beyond his ability to respond adequately to. Children with this kind of sensitivity may know someone is ill before anyone else does. They may know that a certain adult can't be trusted. They may know another is sad when no one else spots it. This isn't a mystical, odd perception. These children can understand the knowledge that is in the yin and yang flows. It is simply another way of perceiving. If this reminds you of a sensitive child in your world, validate his or her feelings. Don't deny them the truth with evaluations of your own. You can ask children who are sensitive to further what they feel. Let them know that this way of perceiving is valuable. You may not change your mind about Janie, but you can value their different opinion and how they arrived at it, mysterious though it may be.

You can also have a lot of fun cross-referencing with children. For example:

- What is Auntie Annie's texture? (Prickly, soft, spongy, rough, and so on?)
- What color is Lauren today? (Orange, pink, black?)
- What is Rufus (the dog) saying right now?

- What color is the day?
- What texture are you today?
- How much space does your energy take up today?

To a child who has energy intelligence, questions such as these open up a world of eloquent communication between the two of you. If your child is enjoying it, ask questions like, "When Auntie Annie is pink, how will she behave?" Let your own imagination run free. This game is fun, and soon you'll both be laughing with the joy of it.

Often energetically sensitive children feel overly stimulated or emotionally over the top. This is because they don't keep others' energies at bay. They actually take them to themselves quite personally. This is the source of their great sensitivities, a marvelous strength in life, but also the source of their lack of complete separation from others. Learning about energy helps them to acknowledge this type of intelligence and feel more at home in the world. Teaching them how to have energy boundaries (these are also good for adults) is useful, too.

One exercise I like is to take some string and make a circle about an arm's length long around yourself or the child. Sit in that circle. Imagine that the circumference of the circle is actually a part of an egg-like shape that surrounds you from top to bottom, completely containing you and in which you have complete freedom of movement and choice. Say out loud, "This is my space. No one enters this space but me. I am safe and secure in my space. I can draw it up to my skin or expand it to fill the room. The choice is mine. This is my space for me alone." This may help define a feeling of contained safety that is often elusive for the energy sensitive child.

CHAPTER 16
Senior Moments

One of the biggest challenges seniors have with T'ai Chi is remembering what to do when. Then, anxiety about doing it right starts to rise, and that complicates the problem even more. T'ai Chi and QiGong provide a perfect opportunity to adapt to your own abilities and still reap the rewards.

Breaking Old Habits and Developing New Ones

Over time, our bodies develop habits. These habits have to do with how we move. It feels normal and right, for example, for someone to have a rigid back if he or she has had it for years. It feels normal for another to hold the hips tight, favoring one side of the body over the other. It feels completely normal and correct to walk in a certain way, twist in a predictable way, carry your heads at a certain angle. These all feel right, even if we are starting to have back problems, walking problems, shoulder aches, and so on.

These habits, of course, all stem from symptoms that all is not well in your body alignment and structural health. It is so much easier, though, to stay with what feels familiar: "I've always moved this way!" "Why should I change?" "If it isn't broken, don't fix it." These are common feelings we may express when trying to learn something new. That much-used cliché, "You can't teach an old dog new tricks" may apply to opinions, personal beliefs, and standards that have been developed—even fought for—in life, but it doesn't really apply to movement.

The trick to creating new muscle memory is to start from where you are. Start with the natural movements in this chapter and your muscle memory will expand. The nervous system thrives on variety—not overload, but variety. In moving in an expanding way, your nervous system experiences a healthy enlivening. You, in turn, feel more alive. As your movement, such as sitting down and standing up, becomes easier and more normal, you will find that your range of ability for doing other simple tasks opens up. For example, your back may loosen from practicing a swinging motion. Because all the muscles of the body are completely intertwined, you may find your reach to the upper shelf to get the jar is simpler, turning in the car to see oncoming traffic is easier, and in general, you feel less stiff. As your muscle memory grows through continued practice of sitting and standing, you may start to wonder whether you can do other exercises. This is your body's natural desire for movement and your nervous system's love of variety joining in to say, "Hey, let's have a little more of this!"

At this point, you can go in a variety of directions. You can extend toward the chair work (see Chapter 17) if your balance isn't great. If your balance is okay (and maybe improving as a result of the sitting and standing), try Chapters 9 and 10 and begin the practices. You're building muscle memory as you break up old body habits of rigidity. Just be sure to take the exercises at your own pace. If T'ai Chi postures are too frustrating, try QiGong. Many people of all ages find this wonderful ancient practice answers their needs perfectly.

Whatever your approach, the result will be that you will have a better range of movement. Your balance will become steadier. Your breath will deepen. Chi will fill your body. These will all create a greater feeling of well-being, and that feeling is so critical as your body ages. When your body starts to develop a life of its own—aching, stiff, and so on—it is scary. It doesn't matter how many people have experienced it before you.

This is the time of life when a feeling of physical well-being is critical. It feels like a golden gift when it is there. Sometimes the feeling is because your physical nature is feeling better. Instead of feeling your health slipping through your fingers, you're improving it. That sense of personal power itself creates well-being. This feeling is also generated by an inner belief that everything is progressing as it should and all is in its right place. This is the spiritual component, and T'ai Chi and QiGong affect them both positively.

Check out Chapter 6 for tips on getting started in your practice. Check your room from the perspective of safety, aesthetics, and light. Do what you can to get your T'ai Chi and QiGong space safe and comfortable for you.

Many seniors have difficulty remembering the sequence of the T'ai Chi form. This can be an unpleasant source of discouragement and can lead some to break off their practice. There are a number of solutions to this problem that allow a person to practice with less memorization:

- Attend a class tailored to seniors or a class that doesn't require precise practice in between class meetings.
- Purchase an easy-to-follow video and practice with it.
- Focus your practice on easier-to-recall drills such as those presented in Chapters 10 and 12.

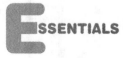 **SSENTIALS**

Many of the benefits in terms of balance, flexibility, increased range of motion, and relaxation available in a more complex T'ai Chi and QiGong practice regime will also be gained through a simpler pattern. In any case, start simply, and if you find this style of exercise rewarding, look into the other avenues.

Trying Senior Exercises

In this section, I include a modification of the Arms Swinging Up and Down QiGong that can be used for standing up and sitting down, as well as a few additional exercises that will help to further improve balance and energy flow.

STANDING UP-SITTING DOWN DRILL

When we were young and filled with energy, we could use our bodies inefficiently and still get the job done. As we've aged, we must get wiser in our energy use. This drill helps you use your momentum to stand up and sit down more easily.

Starting seated, you raise the arms overhead (see **FIGURE 16-1**). Reach forward and down to the floor, allowing the whole trunk to lean forward (see **FIGURE 16-2**).

Roll back up to sitting again. Do this a couple of times until you're comfortable with this portion of the movement. Don't strain; use your momentum. When you're ready for the next part, position your feet close to the chair as you do when preparing to stand, and as you reach to the floor, allow your bottom to lift slightly off the chair as you take your weight into your feet (see **FIGURE 16-3**).

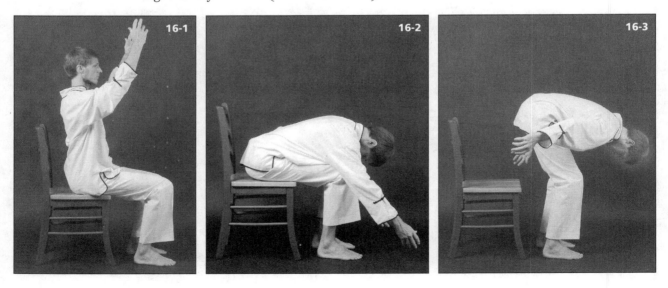

Roll back into the chair again and repeat a couple of times until you're comfortable with this part. For the next part, after you've reached for the floor and then gotten your weight into your feet, push through the soles of the feet by straightening the legs and unroll the whole body to vertical. Allow the arms to swing loosely with the motion until they are overhead (see **FIGURE 16-4**).

To reverse and sit down, reach down and bend your knees in order to replicate the position you were in just before you pushed through the feet to stand. The forward reach allows you to counterbalance with the pelvis reaching for the chair, then the arms swing through behind with their momentum (see **FIGURE 16-5**). Now settle into your chair and roll up to an upright seated position, allowing your arms to swing up above your head once more.

This drill works well with many different kinds of chairs. It is more difficult with low, soft couches and chairs, and very difficult if a table is in the way. Still, practice this on a good chair, and you will find ways to adapt it to less ideal conditions. As you swing through this movement, be sure to allow your head and neck to extend with it (rather than tightening and curling the neck back and up).

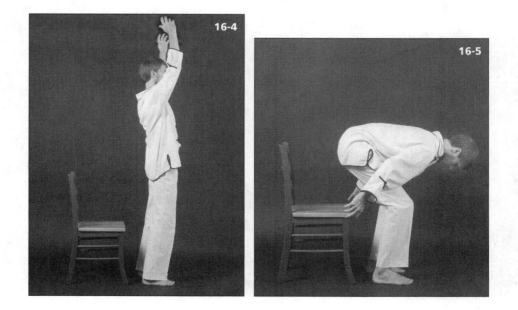

ENERGY BALL PLAY

This exercise works especially well after you've built up the chi in your hands with Holding the Moon or Earth and Heaven QiGong exercises. Stand in a weight 50/50 stance with the feet parallel and hip- to shoulder-width apart. Shift the weight more into the left and hold a ball slightly to the left side with the left hand high (see **FIGURE 16-6**).

Feel the energy between your palms. Shift the weight more into the right and turn the torso slightly to the right rolling the ball upside down so that you're holding it with the right hand above (see **FIGURE 16-7**). Notice the movement of the hips and thighs and be sure not to twist the knees. Relax, breathe deeply, and keep the movement smooth. Do this about fifteen times.

You can also do this energy ball exercise in a 70/30 stance. Start with the left foot forward and hold a ball with the left hand above (see **FIGURE 16-8**).

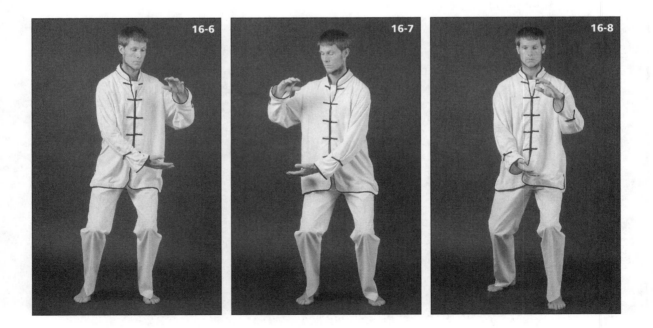

Shift the weight mostly into the right leg and roll the ball so that now the right hand is held above (see **FIGURE 16-9**). Again, notice the movement of the hips and thighs and be sure not to twist the knees. Relax, breathe deeply, and keep the movement smooth. Do this about fifteen times and then do it fifteen times with the other foot forward and that hand above to start.

Moving the lower body in the same kind of way, but adding a step, you can change the way you move the energy ball. This uses the ninety degrees stepping drill described in Chapter 10. Because of the slow, controlled step, this exercise will help your balance. Starting again in a 70/30 stance with the left foot forward, have your left arm in Ward Off and the right Resting on the Pillow of Air. This is the Grasp Sparrow's Tail, Ward Off Left posture (see **FIGURE 16-10**).

Sink fully into the left leg, drawing the right foot in beneath you and hold a ball with the left hand held high (see **FIGURE 16-11**). Then reach out the right foot pointing 90 degrees to the right and a little wide and place it down on the heel (see **FIGURE 16-12**).

As you shift, the pelvis will turn to prevent twisting the knee and the left foot should turn in 45 degrees, rotating on the heel. The right arm

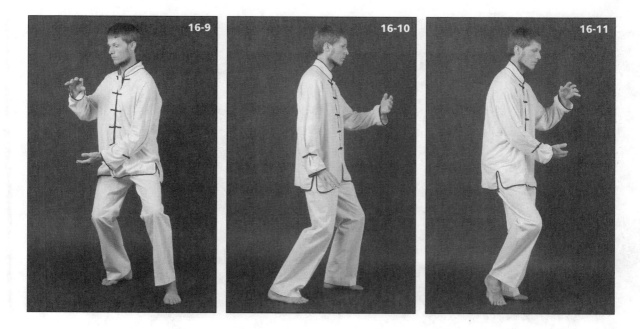

goes into a Ward Off and the left is now Resting on a Pillow of Air. This is the Grasp Sparrow's Tail, Ward Off Right posture with the left hand down (see **FIGURE 16-13**).

Sink fully into the right leg now and draw the left foot in beneath you, scooping the left arm in under the right to hold the ball on the right side. Then reach the left foot out pointing 90 degrees to the left and a little wide and place it down on the heel. As you shift, the pelvis will turn to prevent twisting the knee and the right foot should turn in, rotating on the heel. The left arm goes into a Ward Off and the right is now in Resting on a Pillow of Air. Repeat this exercise about ten times on each side, feeling or imagining the energy between your arms and palms as you stretch it out and hold it in a ball, only to stretch it out once more.

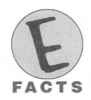

FACTS

Stretching before each T'ai Chi workout helps to prevent injury and promotes the best possible practice. If you're flexible, you'll be free to turn your attention to breathing, position, grace, style, and so on. Flexibility builds upon itself if you incorporate daily stretching. But be gentle and patient. Don't stretch too forcefully, or your muscles will tighten and become sore.

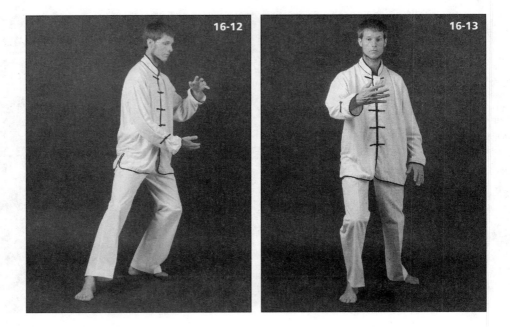

16-12

16-13

CHAPTER 17
Seated T'ai Chi

Seated T'ai Chi is an adaptation of T'ai Chi if you're not steady on your feet or are unable to stand but still want to enjoy the benefits of T'ai Chi and QiGong. Although QiGong and T'ai Chi must be altered when you're confined to a chair, practice can still be quite beneficial. When seated, the function of sitting bones corresponds to that of the feet when standing.

Getting Started

Many of the motions in QiGong and T'ai Chi involve a wavelike motion that begins in the feet and is expressed through the arms and hands. When seated, the wave initiates from your contact with the chair through your sitting bones. Because the distance the wave travels is less and you can't make use of the large muscles of the legs and hips, you must make smaller waves by changing the angle of the pelvis (using the mobility of the spine).

When seated in your chair, set yourself up to be comfortable. For these exercises, if you can, use a stool or a chair with no arms. Sit with your body supported on the sitting bones and stabilized by the feet flat on the floor. Choose a chair height so that your thighs are horizontal or even tilted a little up. Avoid a posture where your thighs tilt down because this tends to strain the lower back. Let your arms and hands rest comfortably on the thighs or in your lap. Make sure your pelvis is a little tilted forward to preserve the natural forward curve of the lower back. **FIGURE 17-1** shows the correct posture, whereas in **FIGURE 17-2**, the lower back is collapsed into a slouch and in **FIGURE 17-3**, the pelvis is tilted too far forward and the back is too arched.

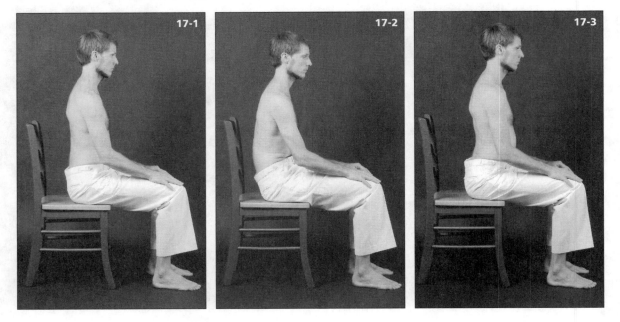

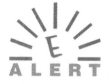

As with all T'ai Chi movements, even when sitting, remember to move in a way that's comfortable and appropriate for you. Be careful not to strain as you practice seated exercises.

Doing Warm-Ups

In this section, I draw on material from Chapter 9 and offer suggestions and modifications for doing these from a chair. Refer back to this chapter, as appropriate.

 CROSS CRAWL

For this one, simply tap the right knee with your left hand, then the left knee with your right hand. Allow your waist to twist with this motion.

 CROSS CRAWL WITH TWIST

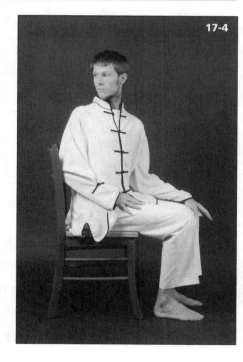

17-4

Modify this warm-up to a simple twist from side to side. Rest your hands on your knees and start by looking from one side to the other as a comfortable twist for the neck. Then slowly increase the twist by drawing your right hand to your right hip as you look to the right. (See **FIGURE 17-4**.)

Keep the spine straight. To make this exercise more intense, bring your forearms up to breast level and increase the speed of the twist. If you can, move your knees up and down with the movement so that as you look and twist to the right, the right knee goes up slightly.

INFINITY ARMS

This one is the same as in Chapter 9. Move your knees up and down with the movement if you can.

 ### SHOULDER ROLLS

This one is the same as in Chapter 9.

 ### HULA PELVIS AND SEXY PELVIS

We blend these two. Sit forward on the chair with your feet flat on the ground and your arms comfortably on your legs. Find the sitting bones of the pelvis and rock in a circle on those bones. Shift your weight to one side and tilt your pelvis back, to the other side, and forward. Go around in circles seven times one way and seven times the other.

 ### FOOT FIGURE EIGHT

If you can lift your foot, twirl it at the ankle seven times in one direction, then seven times in the other. Do it with the other foot also.

WRIST SWIRLS

You drop the leg stretch, but otherwise this exercise is the same as in Chapter 9.

 ### ELBOW MASSAGE

This one is the same as in Chapter 9.

PLIÉ

Drop this exercise altogether.

STRETCHES

Remember, the current research indicates that a maintenance level stretch should be no shorter than ten seconds, while a stretch to increase range of motion must be held for thirty seconds or more. Choose the time you spend in each position accordingly. Many of the stretches described previously involve stretching the legs. These, of course, are hard to do in a chair.

- To Sides: This stretch is the same as in Chapter 9.
- Sun Salutation: We drop this stretch completely.
- Neck: This stretch is the same as in Chapter 9.
- Ankles: This stretch is the same as in Chapter 9.

Performing QiGong Practices

This sections reviews the material from Chapter 12 and offers suggestions and modifications for doing these from a chair. Refer back to that chapter, as appropriate.

 BREATH STIMULATION

This exercise is the same as in Chapter 12.

 MERIDIAN STIMULATION

This exercise is the same as in Chapter 12.

HOLDING THE MOON FULL-BODY BREATHING

This exercise is the same as in Chapter 12—see **FIGURE 17-5**.

EARTH AND HEAVEN BREATHING

This exercise is the same as in Chapter 12 except that you drop the action of the legs.

SWIMMING DRAGON

This exercise is the same as in Chapter 12 except that you drop the movement of the legs and the counterbalance occurs from the sitting bones up (see **FIGURE 17-6**).

SPAGHETTI ARMS WITH WEIGHT SHIFT

You change this to a twisting drill in which you start with the hands on the thighs and simply turn your head and look first in one direction, then the other. Then as you look over the right shoulder, slide your right hand to your hip so that the twist goes into the whole torso. Then look over the left shoulder, sliding your right hand toward your knee and your left hand to your left hip. This movement is similar to part of the Cross Crawl with Twist exercise described earlier in this chapter (refer to **FIGURE 17-4**), but here your focus is on coordinating your breath with the movement. Inhale as you twist one way, exhale as you twist the other way. Repeat this about ten times on each side.

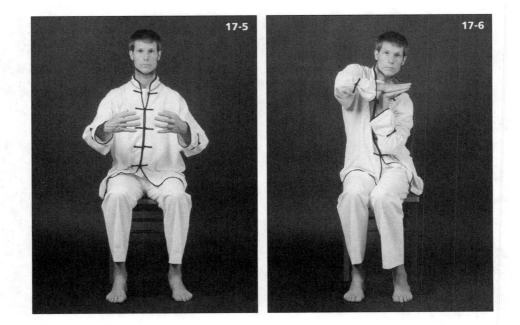

17-5   17-6

ARM SWINGING UP AND DOWN

This exercise is the same as in Chapter 12 except that as the arms go down and back, you bend at the waist. Start with the arms overhead (see **FIGURE 17-7**), and then bend at the waist as you reach down toward the floor (see **FIGURE 17-8**), allowing the momentum of your arms to swing them behind you.

Then push through the feet and uncoil the torso, bringing your arms overhead again. Exhale going down and inhale going up. Start with only a few repetitions of this one and be gentle because it may be hard on your back muscles.

CLEANSING WALK

For this exercise, drop the walking part but use the same arm motion (as in Chapter 12) of gathering energy and settling it down each side.

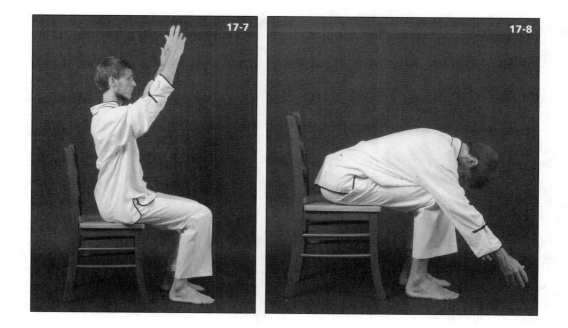

WU CHI

This exercise is modified from Chapter 12 into a seated meditation. Sit with your body supported on the sitting bones and stabilized by the feet flat on the floor. Choose a chair height so that your thighs are horizontal or even tilted a little up. Avoid a posture where your thighs tilt down because this tends to strain the lower back. Let your arms and hands rest comfortably on your thighs or in your lap. Make sure that the pelvis is a little tilted forward to preserve the natural forward curve of your lower back.

Lightly extend the spine through the crown of your head, shoulders resting on the rib cage and the rib cage mobile with the breath. Let your tongue lightly touch the roof of your mouth and allow your neck to be free and your head to float with your chin slightly tucked. After you're in your Wu Chi, bring looseness to your joints by breathing deeply and bringing the movement of your breath into the whole body. From the outside, you should appear to be sitting still, but from the inside, you should feel your whole body mobile with the breath.

 ROCKING ON THE BALLS OF THE FEET

Drop this exercise altogether.

Practicing T'ai Chi Basics

This section reviews the material from Chapters 10 and 11 and offers suggestions and modifications for doing these movements from a chair. Refer to these chapters, as appropriate. For this section, refer to the photos of how the movements are done when standing, but you're dropping all the stances and stepping patterns while the arm and hand movements remain the same.

Remember that in adapting these exercises to a chair, you make a fundamental modification: You are no longer turning fully from one direction to another and you eliminate the momentum from shifting your weight and turning your waist. Instead, the power for these movements arises primarily from your ability to twist through the length of the spine while still remaining stable on your chair. As you twist to the right, you create the ability to twist strongly to the left and to direct this momentum through your arms. In addition, in movements such as Withdraw and Push, you also make use of a subtle vertical wave through the spine.

One of the most important foundations of relaxed movement is making sure that you stay within your comfort range. As you twist from side to side, don't twist so far that you're uncomfortable or start to lose your sense of connection with the earth through your sitting bones, the chair, or your feet. When your hands are in front of you, don't reach past the line of your knees. Allow your neck and your gaze to turn with your twists.

PREPARATION, WU CHI

Start in your seated Wu Chi as described in the preceding section of this chapter.

BEGINNING, LIFTING HANDS

Exhale and allow your shoulders to become a little concave, initiating forward momentum in your arms. Inhale and support that momentum, raising the arms up, palms drooping down at the wrists, until they are slightly lower than the shoulders. Exhale and straighten the wrists, and, allowing the elbows to settle downward, bring the wrists back toward the shoulders in a Begging Dog posture. Inhale and straighten the wrists, fingers to the sky. Exhale and settle the energy down the right and left sides of the body with the hands going down to the sides to rest on Pillows of Air.

GRASP SPARROW'S TAIL, WARD OFF LEFT

Inhale as you raise both arms to thigh height and then twist slightly to the right, creating a ball held on the right side with the right hand high, left hand low. Exhale as you settle the right arm down to rest on a Pillow of Air and the left arm expands forward into a left Ward Off with the palm facing the center of the chest at about the level of the bottom of the breast bone (see **FIGURE 17-9**).

GRASP SPARROW'S TAIL, WARD OFF RIGHT

Inhale as you twist slightly to the left holding a ball vertically with the left hand held high. Exhale as you push and roll this ball to the front, ending up with the palms facing each other horizontally as if you were holding a soccer ball. The left hand is close to the body.

GRASP SPARROW'S TAIL, ROLLBACK

Inhale, twisting slightly to the right. Your right arm extends a bit to the corner while your left palm turns to face your right elbow. Exhale as you twist to the left, drawing your hands toward your left hip. You end holding a diagonal ball with the right hand on top.

GRASP SPARROW'S TAIL, PRESS

Inhale, turning and raising the ball at the left side so that your left hand ends up on top. Exhale and squeeze the ball until your left palm presses against the right with your left palm closer to the body, hands on the midline at mid-chest level.

GRASP SPARROW'S TAIL, PUSH

Inhale as your left hand presses through the right, and your hands separate to shoulder width and withdraw to just in front of your shoulders, palms facing away. Exhale as you push the hands away at the same level. (See **FIGURE 17-10**.)

SINGLE WHIP

Inhale as you twist to the right, ending up holding a vertical ball to the right side with your right hand high. Close your right hand into a Hook Hand. Exhale as you extend your hooked right hand to the right rear corner while you also bring your left forearm in an upward diagonal across your chest and then turn your palm away to do a one-handed push with your left hand. (See **FIGURE 17-11**.) The movement of your right and left arms should counterbalance each other in timing and power.

LIFT HANDS, OPEN/CLOSE

Inhale and spread your arms open in a welcoming embrace, facing forward. Exhale and close your arms to the midline. Move your arms slightly down and up to engage the shoulder muscles of your back (the latissimus dorsi). The left palm ends facing your right elbow with a few inches of space between.

SHOULDER STROKE

Inhale and Roll Back to the left side, ending with a diagonal ball near the left hip with the right hand held high. Exhale and press the left hand to your right wrist, creating a feeling of extending energy forward through the right forearm. The line of the forearm points down 45 degrees. Keep the right forearm within five inches of the front of your body.

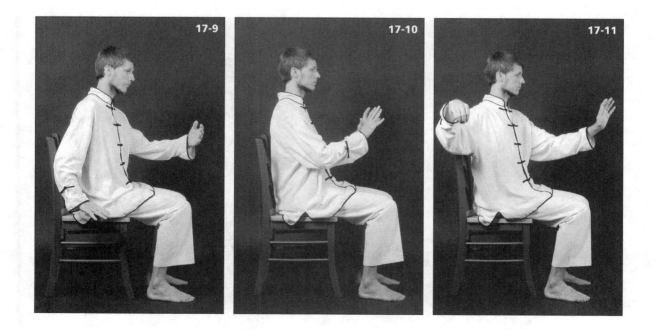

17-9   17-10   17-11

WHITE CRANE SPREADS WINGS

Inhale and float your still-connected arms up to solar plexus height (area of the belly just below the sternum) at the midline. Exhale, twisting slightly to the right while you extend your left arm down to the left of your knees while your right arm extends up to the right. Both arms end up in arc shapes, the left with the palm down at mid-calf height; the right a bit higher than the temple with the palm facing slightly up to the right corner. (See **FIGURE 17-12**.) This is one of the few postures where your elbow (in this case, the right elbow) is higher than your shoulder.

 ## BRUSH KNEE AND TWIST

Inhale as you drop your right elbow and raise your left hand as your arm moves across the body to the right so that you're holding a diagonal ball with your left hand high (see **FIGURE 17-13**). Drop your left arm palm down and raise your right palm up near the right shoulder. Exhale as you sweep your left arm across to the left just above your lap, fingertips at your knee, and execute a single-handed push with your right hand, the first knuckle of the thumb ending up on the centerline, the fingertips just lower than your shoulder.

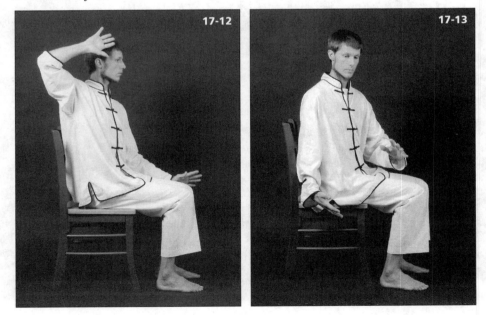

17-12

17-13

PLAY LUTE

Inhale, twisting a little to the left so that your right arm reaches forward as your left arm settles downward. Exhale as you twist back and a little to the right, drawing your right arm back and extending your left arm forward so that your hand is on the midline. Your left palm faces to the right and is about as high as your solar plexus. Your right palm faces the left elbow with three to four inches between.

BRUSH KNEE AND TWIST

Inhale as you drop your right elbow and move your left hand across your body to the right so that you're holding a diagonal ball with your left hand high. Drop your left arm palm down and raise your right palm up near your right shoulder. Exhale as you sweep your left arm across to the left just above your lap, fingertips at knee, and execute a single-handed push with your right hand, the first knuckle of your thumb ending up on the centerline, the fingertips just lower than the shoulder.

STEP FORWARD, DEFLECT DOWNWARD, PARRY AND PUNCH

Inhale longer than usual, twisting slightly to the left holding a low horizontal ball with your right hand further forward. Turn the right palm up and make a fist while circling the left arm up, hand near your ear. Twist to the right. Your left arm reaches forward on the midline, while your right fist arcs up across the chest and withdraws to the right hip. The movement and timing of the arms counterbalance each other. Exhaling, draw your left hand back on the left side of the midline and punch forward with your right. The fist finishes in a vertical position, just to the right of the midline, at solar plexus height.

WITHDRAW AND PUSH

Inhaling, extend your right arm a bit to the left corner and reach under your right elbow with your left palm up. Twist to the right and draw your right arm back across the top of your left wrist. Form a horizontal ball at solar plexus height to the right side. Exhaling, twist back to the center and execute a two-handed push.

APPARENT CLOSE UP AND CROSS HANDS

Inhale, opening your chest and circling your arms out and down until they are palm up above your thighs. Exhale, crossing below your wrists with the left on top and extend your arms in an upward diagonal until your fingertips are shoulder high. Your arms are still crossed a little below the wrists.

 COMPLETE

Inhale, separating your arms, palms up, to shoulder width. Exhale, rolling the hands over, thumbs inward, and settling your palms to your beginning sitting posture, hands resting on your thighs. Relax and breathe deeply, feeling the whole body.

Applying Martial Arts (Self-Defense)

In order to more deeply understand the movements of the T'ai Chi form, familiarize yourself with the martial applications of each movement. See Chapter 18 for a more thorough discussion. As is true for standing, the first step in self-defense is to not be on the line of attack. This requires that you identify the line of attack and position yourself to one side. The martial applications require you to identify the line of attack (directed to your midline) and to deflect it to one side or the other. It may be helpful for you to imagine yourself as a cowcatcher on a train or as the bow of a boat. Energy comes toward you, and by creating a diagonal line of defense off to one side or the other, you guide the energy to the side and away. In some ways, it is easier to see this dynamic when the movements are done from the chair.

Practicing Push-Hands

Two-person practices (discussed in Chapter 13) are quite difficult to do while seated simply because it is more difficult for two seated people to be within each other's reach. However, it is worth the trouble to try this even if only to get the feel for applying these practices with another person. Start by facing each other with your chairs as close as possible. You can also experiment with sitting beside one another. The stationary two-person practices described in Chapter 13 can be easily adapted to this structure.

As with the standing drills, the key is to follow your partner's motion (as opposed to blocking or resisting it) in order to build your sensitivity and flexibility.

T'ai Chi has opened up a whole new world for me, and as a wheelchair-bound person, a whole new confidence in myself. T'ai Chi brings a good health benefit. I'm not a very strong person, but the gentle rhythm and movements help exercise my muscles, help circulation, and help teach me to breathe properly and to relax. No matter what your strength is, you can benefit by learning T'ai Chi, even if you can only do parts of it.

When I started, my stress level was high and I always held my shoulders up, which felt normal to me. With practice and my instructor regularly reminding me of the position of my shoulders, it became natural to keep them down, which dropped my daily pain level. You may get a similar benefit.

When you're learning T'ai Chi, you also learn the techniques for protection. You learn to let your attacker, or something harmful, into your space, where you have more control. This makes it easier for a wheelchair-bound person or a person needing an aiding device to protect him- or herself. It was hard for me to practice this and let someone get that close to me, but now I feel safer in crowds and enjoy my time out more.

Thank you for giving me the opportunity to share my love for T'ai Chi in this book!

—Terry E. Wright

CHAPTER 18

Practicing Self-Defense with T'ai Chi

Historically, T'ai Chi was used for martial arts and was called T'ai Chi Ch'uan. Although self-defense is not the focus of Western T'ai Chi, it is important to demonstrate the full range of life to which T'ai Chi relates. It is becoming more and more relevant to have some good basic tools for self-defense, and this chapter gets you started.

Sharpening Skills to Resolve Conflicts

Along with sharpening your tools for physical action to defense, other tools can also be useful. These tools can be found in conflict resolution classes and books. It is also useful to sharpen up your communication skills. Remarkably, many of your conflicts are simply a matter of not communicating with personal clarity and empathy for the other person. You can likely find excellent classes and books that share tools for shifting your routine communication to a more effective method whenever the situation requires it. A method called Giraffe Communication by Marshall Risenfield is quite useful (check any Internet search engine for details). You can probably find many others, as well.

Getting Ready to Defend Yourself

The following sections get you in the proper mindset to learn the specific forms.

Being Prepared Through Perception and T'ai Chi Practice

The martial applications of T'ai Chi are based on the fundamental philosophy that in order to maintain balance and your ability to influence events in an unpredictable world, you must first understand what is happening. You gain understanding by paying close attention. Only after you understand the truth of what is occurring are you able to interact with it wisely. To gain accurate perception, you tune your body to be a sensitive instrument. Doing so requires knowing ourselves so well that we can distinguish between our own internal filters or noise and what is happening outside us. For example, if I know I have a phobia of snakes, I can modulate my own distress over my child playing with a garter snake. Just because my body gets upset about it doesn't mean it's actually dangerous.

Become streetwise by knowing the danger level in your community. And if danger lurks, pick the safest times to venture out. If you live in a risky area, you know what needs to be done, so I won't go on.

T'ai Chi can help if you're surprised by practicing some reactions well in advance of a treacherous situation. Find a friend and go through the instructions in this chapter. Do it enough that you have a muscle memory for the action. Should you ever need it, the skills will be in this muscle memory and may help at that critical moment.

T'ai Chi requires fully opening, relaxing, and enlivening each joint and increasing the sensitivity and vitality of the body—these are training byproducts but are the primary reason most people study T'ai Chi. You achieve these byproducts not only by focusing on them, but by carefully practicing the movements, especially with a partner. It is difficult to practice the movements of T'ai Chi with precision without the martial component because they lose their context and become vague.

Seeing Martial Arts as a Metaphor

For most people, conflicts are primarily of an interpersonal nature involving words and deeds far more than physical battle. Any good martial arts or self defense approach must serve as a metaphor that is equally applicable to these daily conflicts. By practicing the T'ai Chi responses in this chapter, building your sensitivity to yourself and others, you can become increasingly able to see the truth in any situation and choose how best to respond.

For many, the superficial understanding of martial arts is that you train to be able to hit any energy that comes toward you. Indeed, some beginning levels of martial training use this approach. This is a very limited training method, however, and certainly doesn't translate very well to daily use in relationships. A well-balanced self-defense philosophy should work well whether applied to intimate or business relationships, physical conflict or the freeway. Ultimately, all martial arts mature to the understanding that we need to identify the energy coming toward us before we hit it. T'ai Chi places an early emphasis on using the whole body and mind to understand the truth of a situation.

As a consequence, martial applications in T'ai Chi make use of the arms and hands first as sensory organs and secondly as weapons. The first part of a martial application entails receiving the other person's attack enough to understand its structure—only then do you counter. Ideally, the momentum of the attack is directly transferred back in the counter whether through a simple twist or by allowing the attack to compress the joints of the body as springs, which are then released in the counter.

Understanding the Intent—and the Consequences— of Self-Defense

The intention in martial applications is not nice. My hope is that you will never have to use these practices. As you explore this material, however, recognize that you have three levels of response available to you, and these should be based on your attacker's intent:

- Your "attacker" is a fellow student—be gentle, but firm enough so that you can both feel what's going on.
- Your attacker is easily discouraged—deliver enough pain or humiliation to make him or her pause and then run away.
- Your attacker is intent on hurting or killing you or yours—pull out the stops and incapacitate him or her and then run away!

Understand that the movements that follow aren't the only martial applications, but these will get you started. More serious students should study with a competent instructor and read other books to expand your understanding. Ultimately, you want to move beyond set martial applications into a more free and personal expression of your will.

ESSENTIALS

To practice at this level, the student must pay attention to the martial applications of the movements and must practice Push-Hands (see Chapter 13). Transmitting power requires fully understanding your own body and the possibilities within it, while discerning the target requires delicately sensing your opponent, and both can be learned through Push-Hands. Keep in mind, however, that these skills are not all that are required in order to be effective at self-defense.

Performing the Movements

Take the action movements in this section one step at a time. Let the movements sink gently into the muscles and the memory of your body. In order to correctly practice the form, use the martial applications to help you move your body more precisely by visualizing your opponent and the purpose of your movements. If you can, enlist a friend when practicing these applications so that you can really get a feel for them. Do the interactions gently and slowly and remember to use your limbs to feel the nature of the incoming attack even as you deflect it. If you would rather practice with a group, check out your neighborhood YMCA or martial arts center. They may offer beginner classes in self-defense.

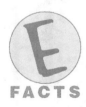

FACTS

Adding emotional centering to your T'ai Chi practice requires that you address any confusion about the sequences so that you can go through the movements without that stress, do your form slowly to draw out your breathing to switch on the "rest and repose" sympathetic nervous system, keep your attention in the present to reduce mental chatter and eliminate worry, and practice at least daily, because emotional stability is more easily lost than physical fitness.

My thanks to student Ann Ramage for posing with Fernando on these attacks. Although she doesn't look like a classic mugger, you never know!

LIFTING HANDS

In **FIGURE 18-1**, we are grabbed from behind in a bear hug. To do this, allow you partner to really get a solid hold on you. He or she should be pinning your elbows.

CREATING SPACE

To get clear of a bear hug, bend your knees and extend through your arms as in the beginning of lifting hands (see **FIGURE 18-2**). As you sink down through your legs and raise the upper arms, your leverage will be greater than your opponent's, and your elbows will become free. At this point you can counter with a variety of moves, one of the simplest being to shift to one side and jam your elbow into your opponent's solar plexus (the area of the belly just below the sternum). You could also stomp down, dragging the side of your foot down your attacker's shin and then crushing his or her instep.

GRABBED FROM THE SIDE

This application occurs as you start Ward Off Left. Here, you are grabbed from behind on the right side (see **FIGURE 18-3**).

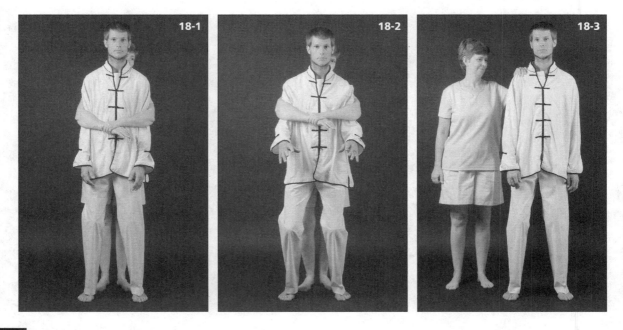

Your opponent may be preparing to hit, knife or shoot you or maybe a friend, so the first step is to look and see! Looking initiates a twist to the right, which you do while shifting into the left leg to help pull out of your attacker's grasp. This gives you an opportunity to gauge your distance, as well.

TURN AND STRIKE

For this position, you hold a ball with your right arm high, placing your elbow in position to strike to your opponent's solar plexus (see **FIGURE 18-4**). You may also use the right arm to help deflect an incoming punch.

WARD OFF LEFT

Here, you intercept an incoming fist with your right hand (see **FIGURE 18-5**). Your opponent steps in with the right and punches to the face with the right. You circle the right hand left then rise to the right as you shift your weight left to be off the line of attack. This is the beginning of Ward Off Left.

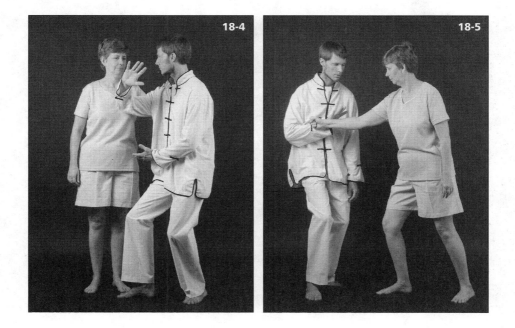

STEP IN

Having deflected and captured the incoming punch, you shift back into the right, freeing the left leg to step forward. The right hand pulls back and down toward the right hip (into the Resting on the Pillow of Air form) while you carry the left arm with the forward momentum of the step to attack under the opponent's arm with your forearm (see **FIGURE 18-6**). After the punch is deflected and the weight is in the right leg, there is a moment of freedom where you can decide upon the appropriate intensity of your counterattack.

WARD OFF RIGHT

In this movement, you're deflecting and capturing a right kick (see **FIGURE 18-7**). Your opponent kicks to the groin with the right leg. Shifting into the left to close the groin with the leg, you further protect the groin and capture his or her foot with your right hand.

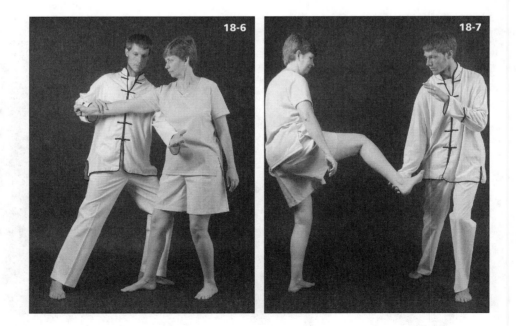

18-6   18-7

LIFT AND PUSH THE LEG AWAY

Stepping toward your opponent with your right foot, you raise her foot with your right hand while pushing it into her with the left hand (see **FIGURE 18-8**). If this is done strongly in practice, your training partner will fall on her tailbone and may strike her head, so be careful!

CAPTURE AND DRAW A LEFT PUNCH DOWN TO THE LEFT

This movement allows you to swallow a left punch. From Ward Off Right, you turn a bit to the right to get your right hand to the outside of your opponent's incoming left punch to the chest or head. Your left hand captures her fist; your right hand is on her elbow. (See **FIGURE 18-9**.)

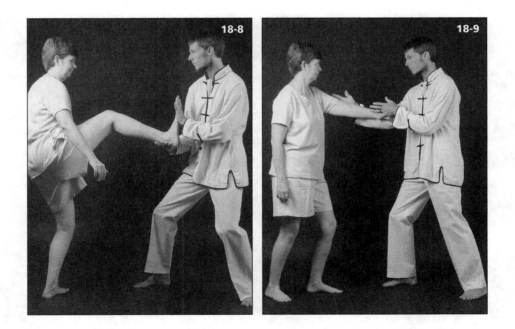

ROLL BACK

Shifting back into the left leg, you draw your opponent's left arm down and to your side, twisting it so that the elbow is up (see **FIGURE 18-10**).

By pushing down on the elbow and drawing up on the wrist or fist, you can either lever your opponent into the dirt or hyperextend and break the elbow. Make sure that you have good control over both the fist and elbow and that the opponent's arm is extended (see **FIGURE 18-11**).

HANDS SEPARATING, SHIFTING BACK

Clear the neck attack after a Press, shifting back and separating your opponent's hands. This move is used to protect from a front grab to the neck or from a two-handed push. As you shift the weight back and separate your opponent's arms to either side, you create an opening for you to go for his or her neck (see **FIGURE 18-12**). If you are subtle, your retreat may cause your opponent to topple a bit toward you. As you come into the opening (see **FIGURE 18-13**), you choose your target: chest, neck, or solar plexus.

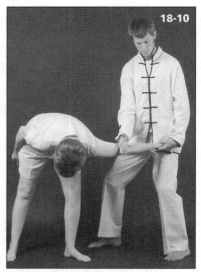

18-10

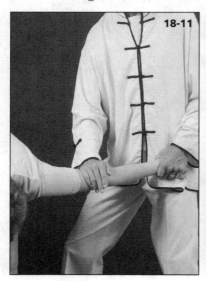

18-11

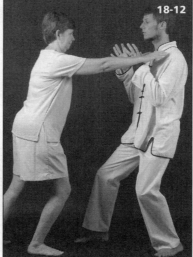

18-12

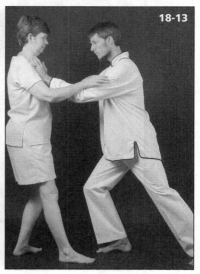

18-13

SINGLE WHIP

As your opponent punches with the left, you capture it with the right and extend it to the right rear—see **FIGURE 18-14**.

Then stepping in with the left leg, you attack with a one-handed push (see **FIGURE 18-15**). If your opponent attacks with the right arm as well, you use your rising left arm to deflect the attack and then come in with the push.

LIFT HANDS OR OPEN AND CLOSE

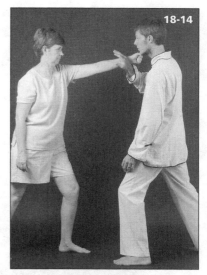

18-14

After a Single Whip (see the preceding section), you open the arms providing your opponent a clear target. He or she punches with the left. (See **FIGURE 18-16**.)

Swinging your arms in, you stabilize her punch between the left palm and right elbow while slapping your opponent's elbow to hyperextend or break it (see **FIGURE 18-17**). If you choose, you can follow that with Roll Back to the left as done in the beginning of the Shoulder Stroke, taking her down to the ground as in **FIGURE 18-10**.

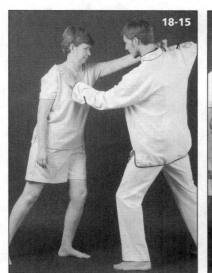

18-15

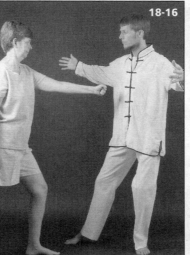

18-16

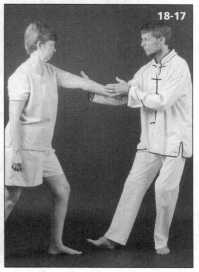

18-17

SHOULDER STROKE

Given an opening, you collide with the opponent's sternum with the deltoid muscle of the upper arm (see **FIGURE 18-18**). Be sure not to lean, because this will lead you to strike with the joint space where the upper arm meets the shoulder socket. If you can't reach with the shoulder, extend the left arm to strike with the heel of the palm to the neck or face (see **FIGURE 18-19**).

 WHITE CRANE

When your opponent pushes, you grasp his or her wrists (see **FIGURE 18-20**). Here, as you receive the opponent's push, you sink into the right leg and grasp the opponent's wrists.

With a knee or kick to the groin, you stretch out your opponent by raising your right hand and sinking your left (see **FIGURE 18-21**). You use your opponent's weight to stabilize yourself and knee or kick him or her in the groin with the left leg.

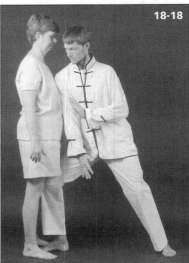

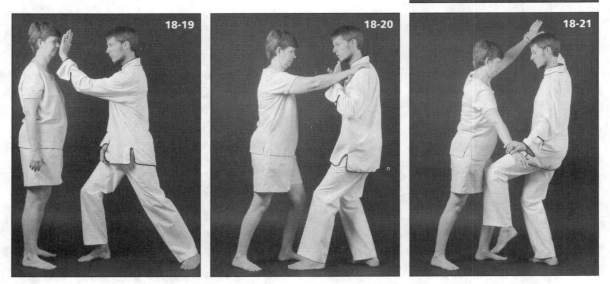

BRUSH KNEE

Here, your opponent kicks with the left leg, and you intercept it with your left hand (see **FIGURE 18-22**). As your opponent kicks with the left, you step in and deflect it past with your left arm.

As your opponent falls into the failed kick, you deliver a one-handed push with the right hand (see **FIGURE 18-23**). This can easily knock your partner over, so when practicing, be careful!

INTERCEPT A LEFT PUNCH, CLOSE AND PUSH

This movement can be done in response to a punch—you simply raise the level of the deflecting hand (see **FIGURE 18-24**).

DEFLECT DOWNWARD, PARRY AND PUNCH

The Back Fist as done here (see **FIGURE 18-25**) can be used to strike downward on the bridge of the nose or the cheekbone.

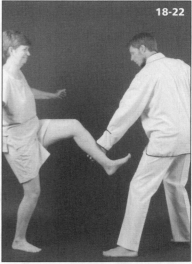

18-22

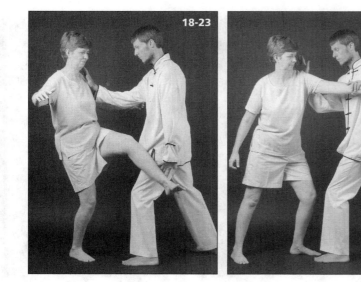

18-23

18-24

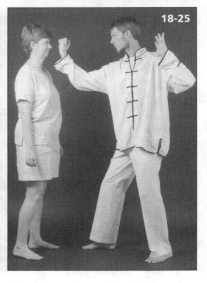

18-25

PUNCH

In the Punch, you reach your left hand out first to grab your opponent and then pull him or her in toward you as you punch. (See **FIGURE 18-26**.)

CROSS HANDS TO CAPTURE AN OVERHAND STRIKE

In Cross Hands, you use crossed hands to locate and capture a strike descending downwards—see **FIGURE 18-27**.

ROLL BACK

Rather than blocking the strike, here you yield to its momentum and reposition your feet to be able to execute a Roll Back to break the arm or throw the opponent into the dirt. (See **FIGURE 18-28**.)

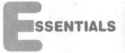

T'ai Chi demonstrates that force—or at least brute force—is not the essential component in self-protection and fighting. A fragile person who is accomplished in T'ai Chi can effectively defend against a strong person. A lot of strength is still needed, but that strength comes from being balanced, relaxed, and focused.

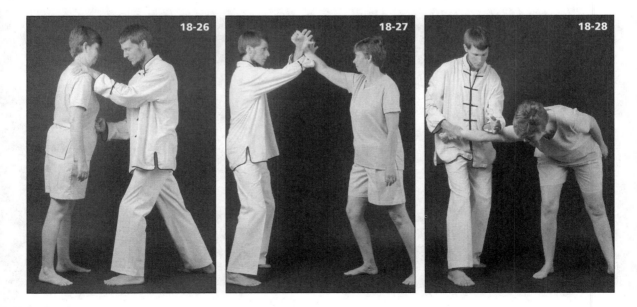

CHAPTER 19

Meditation, Spirituality, and T'ai Chi and QiGong

Does the word "meditation" bring to mind someone sitting cross-legged, hands in lap, eyes closed, with a relaxed body? This commonly seen form is done by millions of people worldwide. Meditation has a variety of forms and techniques, but all are aimed at inner reflection. This is essential for understanding your true nature, instead of the nature created by your habits and your surrounding culture.

Understanding the Seven Basic Meditation Practices

You can find many different forms and techniques of meditation, and all are aimed at the same goal—enlightenment. Enlightenment is defined as attainment of spiritual light. These various techniques are broken down into distinct types of meditation, each one a different path to the same eventual outcome. Because people vary so much, these differences allow everyone to find meditation practices that they are comfortable with:

- Breathing exercises
- Concentrating one's thoughts on one point (QiGong)
- Visualization (art, music, mandalas)
- Mantric yoga (reciting certain words)
- Absorbing one's mind in goodwill or devotional thoughts
- Identifying the mind essence
- Movement and philosophies (yoga, T'ai Chi, QiGong, dance)

Mixing Meditation and Prayer

Meditation and some types of prayer are essentially the same. Some prayers acknowledge the greatness of a higher power; others thank that power for life and gifts; still others ask for intercession in personal or life events.

Another aspect of prayer is the entering into spiritual communion. It is this later form that has the same focus as meditation. Some sitting practices involve different positions of hands: Some use chanting, some use a mantra.

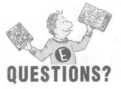

QUESTIONS?

What is a mantra?
A mantra is a simple, powerful phrase repeated over and over throughout the meditation. The words of the mantra are considered to be of essential importance. "Om Mani Padma Hum" is a very common one. In prayer it might be, "I am love." These mantras can also be repeated within as an inner voice as the practitioner goes through daily life.

Practicing Moving Meditation

Another type of meditation is a moving meditation. This is just what it sounds like: The person moves. The movement assists in maintaining a meditative state of mind. One style of this type of meditation is a walking meditation. In this style, the breath is coordinated with the movement of walking, the eyes remain in an unstrained, even gaze, blinking softly. The focus of the mind and thoughts is to direct more and more fully the movements of the body. The body relaxes more deeply into the familiar movement of walking. As a result of this increasing relaxation, the breath/chi moves more fully into the body on ever-deepening breaths.

ESSENTIALS

The mind thought/body/chi/breath union creates an environment of awareness in which the practitioner becomes more and more relaxed, receptive, and alive to the present moment—not relaxed and receptive in the sense of being like a zombie, but in the sense that all the exquisite, finely tuned aspects of life become more clear, more precious, and much more varied.

This ability to see life in this way allows the emergence of one's true nature as his or her habitual nature recedes. The habitual nature is the one we have developed over years of coping with life's stresses and difficult lessons. It is this habitual nature that denies your true nature the opportunity to engage life as a beautiful treasure. The habitual nature negotiates with life, always struggling in some way with fear. All meditation techniques are crafted to bring the true nature forward as the habitual nature recedes. A meditation may be sitting or moving, but the intent is always to become more present by harmonizing the body, mind, and chi.

Movement meditation is perfect for anyone who likes to move, is task-oriented, and gets bored easily. The moving aspects can offset the restlessness that occurs from these personality characteristics. It is often much easier for an action-oriented person to master meditation in movement. The sitting aspects of meditation can be very unrewarding. Each type of meditation has equal value. Find the one that works for you.

And as long as you are doing T'ai Chi and QiGong, the movement aspects of meditation will be a part of your life.

If you already meditate or do communing prayer, you may be concerned that adding T'ai Chi would be too much of a good thing. I do think that would be possible if this was all T'ai Chi and QiGong did; that is, if they were simply a moving meditation. But T'ai Chi and QiGong are so much more than meditation, as this book demonstrates.

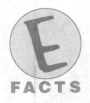

FACTS

Meditation is when theory livens personal knowledge so that the mind is supreme over the body. Through meditation, the mind can transform you. For movement meditation, do the following:

1. Relax.
2. Know emptiness and fullness.
3. Have slowness and evenness.
4. Balance.
5. Root and sink.
6. Breathe.
7. Concentrate.

Harmonizing the Mind and Body

It is the same symphony of body, mind, and breath that T'ai Chi students and teachers are striving for. Stress occurs when the body is doing one thing and the mind is doing another—for example, the body is relaxing in a chair while the thoughts or feelings are engaged in a suspenseful book, movie, or TV show. The body takes on the thought and feeling experience, feeling the stress, anxiety, and concerns generated by the thoughts and feelings as you remain absorbed in the movie, but the body is just sitting. The body, meanwhile, is burdened with unrealized stress responses, extra adrenaline, shortness of breath, and jumpiness.

Even in sleep, the body will not completely discharge this stress. The next day the person may bounce into the day, ready to go at it, and notice that his or her body seems tired. "Late night, probably." Probably not.

When the body and mind are not joined in a creative expressive interaction, the body takes the first hit in the reduced vitality and early aging. The mind takes a later hit by having the sluggishness of the body finally slow it down, too.

This certainly doesn't mean you need to give up your relaxing pleasures. Instead, you can relax while cooking, engaging in a favorite sport focus, or designing or building something. These are activities in which the mind and body are a bit more united in a single process and effort, with the body moving to support the requests of the mind. Even in these events, the mind may still jump to another subject—maybe just for a nanosecond, but that's enough to break the meditation.

A favorite meditation technique that requires nothing more than you and your life is to fully engage in whatever you are doing: washing dishes, walking, talking, silence, or anything else. It is this ability to engage in full presence with the simplest of activities that brings us more spiritual awareness of our true nature and disengages us from our more fearful habitual self. This full awareness in everyday activities sounds easy, but try it. Take some dishes and wash them for five minutes, staying completed focused on the task, even your breath, the whole time. It is very hard! It is a good endeavor because it shows how jumpy the mind is. It shows how hard it is to slow the jumpiness and how easy it is to drift from the present physical moment into a mental interlude.

The Power of Thoughts and Feelings

The belief behind uniting the mind and body is that your thoughts are in charge of you. Whatever is in your thoughts is in full control of you at that moment. Your mind is seen as the source of everything known and unknown. Your thoughts are what you pluck from the vastness of your mind to focus and create experiences in your life. Your feelings allow you to see immediately whether you are creating the life you want. Feelings give quality to your life: If you can focus your thoughts, you have more creative control of your feelings because your thoughts generate your feelings.

Most of your thoughts, however, have nothing to do with the activity of the moment. They have to do with the past or the future. As a result, the feeling state isn't stable in the moment, and is constantly being guided by your bouncing mind. You then become unable to respond in the moment appropriately because you are also feeling pressed upon by the other things your thoughts remind you of. Most of your thoughts have nothing to do with whatever you're physically doing. Because your feelings are directed by your thoughts and those thoughts are bouncing here and there, your feelings are not stable, either. Your feelings then have little to do with whatever is happening at the moment.

Feelings are seldom a pure reaction to the moment. More often, they are greatly influenced by thoughts going somewhere else and influencing your feelings. For example, suppose you've had a hard, long day and someone did something that got under your skin. It continues to bother you if you have intrusive thoughts about it. You get home, and your kids are noisy. You tell them to quiet down. You shout. Your intrusive thoughts have directed your feelings because you are still irritated at and thinking about your coworker. Again, most thoughts have nothing to do with the activity of the moment. Usually, you're thinking about what has happened, what might be happening, or what will happen.

All this is unsettling for the body. The body is so deeply influenced by thoughts and feelings, and yet people seldom do anything that directly expresses thoughts or feelings through bodily action. As a result, at a health level your body is always stressed to some degree. Shortness of breath, upset stomach, and heart palpitations are just a very few of the related problems.

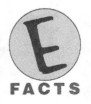

FACTS

A stressed body is not a relaxed body, which is hardly a surprise. But also a tense body can't take in its full amount of breath/chi, and that's a big problem. The body is stressing, responding to all the bouncing thoughts and feelings. Yet this is the scattered-state life that most everyone leads.

The Balance Within and Without

The ancient Chinese believed that God, Love, or the Universe are in the moment, that we are surrounded at all times by this great force of life and love. It is always available to us to show us our true natures and the true nature of life. It is our lack of receptivity that compromises this state of inner fullness and joy. Our receptivity is compromised because we all compromise our ability to simply be here, in this moment.

Because the ancients so deeply believed that any person can find God/Love/Universe within by mastering presence, much time was devoted to cultivating this skill. This is the reason for all the meditation techniques. This is also the reason that T'ai Chi and QiGong facilitate spiritual growth.

ESSENTIALS

The very essence of both T'ai Chi and QiGong is to unite the thoughts, the feelings, and the body to create perfect alignment with the moment. This alignment then draws from Wu Chi, is brought into being with T'ai Chi, and then inspires yin and yang into a balance.

I believe there is no more perfect moving meditation than T'ai Chi and QiGong. T'ai Chi and QiGong are perfectly designed by the ancients to be a moving meditation. If you learn them and continue to practice regularly, even daily, you will understand through your experience the gifts of movement meditation: feeling as though more time is available, being relaxed, breathing easier, and feeling happier.

Instead of leaping in with your first response and then later having second thoughts, you have time to make decisions. Meditation in movement and T'ai Chi specifically create an environment where time becomes more spacious. Life doesn't slow down, there is just more space between events.

As you practice T'ai Chi and make it part of your life, you'll see for yourself what happens. It will happen when you know the QiGong and T'ai Chi well enough that it flows. It will happen when you're practicing in a place you enjoy. It will happen when you start into your practice and your mind, movement, breath, and chi are all there, all in movement, all moving in symphony with one another. Your thoughts will focus. Your feelings will stabilize, and you will be there, opening up to a world yet to be explored, a world of greater harmony, balance, and presence.

One way of describing how this occurs is reviewing Chapter 4. This is the chapter about Wu Chi, T'ai Chi, chi, yin and yang. The great potential/nothingness is brought into movement through intent T'ai chi, and then divided into yin and yang, which are contained in the chi. This T'ai Chi is the energy moment that T'ai Chi (the movement) embodies. This embodiment occurs as you do your T'ai Chi and QiGong practices. You then direct your chi, which holds within it the yin-yang in varying balance in your body and all of life. Your thoughts, feelings, state of health, life experiences, and quality of life are all guided by your personal balance of yin and yang.

Meditation As Body Care

It is in this dynamic moment, when energy moves into the physical, that meditation also rests. Meditation provides a place in inner life where the soul and the body live in harmony. This is not an easy balance to achieve. The life of the body is completely concerned with survival, reproduction, and being included in the group. The life of your spirit, filled with chi, wants to experience life and its changes. The spirit longs for wisdom as a result of growth generated by life and life's experiences. So with the body saying, "I survive and play by those rules," the spirit saying, "I experience and grow, and wisdom is mine," you end up having two very different agendas. This tension between the body's need for security and the spirit's need to experience new challenges is a big problem. This tension can create personal confusion about how to achieve treasured goals. This tension can create illness, stress, early aging, and lack of joy in ordinary existence. This struggle is core in human existence. It is true for everyone—rich or poor, healthy or not, male and female, people in all walks of life. It is this tension that moves through all ethnic and economic groups, creating a common ground for the powerful and powerless. It is life's great leveler.

The ancients' ideal was caring for the body's needs for security with a wise and supportive structure—predictable meals, predictable sleep, no sudden changes, letting the chi flow deeply into the body's tissues. Caring for the spirit was to understand the true nature of one's self, to trust life as the great teachers, to uphold one's personal quality no matter what life brought, and to seek to elevate all of life by expressing personal standards in life. It was the union of these two "maintenance" programs that allowed the ancients to begin to see the wonder of a life lived with body and spirit balanced. A world opened with a change of perspective, giving refined wisdom on how to improve the quality of life for each person alive and in doing so elevate the quality of standards for the group. The work was seen as needing to be done inwardly. The belief was that to change one's self in these ways would produce great, wise appreciation and love of life. It would also change others around this individual and eventually, life improvements would evolve. Meditation was seen as the key to this, that these finer ways of being were impossible to achieve without it. It is the Eastern philosophies' bottom line.

ESSENTIALS

In meditation, the tension between the body's need to survive and the spirit's need to grow in new ways is diminished. This shows itself in reduced body stress, reduction of illness, and slowing of aging.

CHAPTER 20

Feng Shui and
Your T'ai Chi Space

To understand Feng Shui, explore chi from the perspective of it being an all-encompassing force. Chi is an energy flow that links everything in the universe together, including us. Without chi, the liveliness of life ceases. The fuller the chi, the livelier and healthier is the person, animal, plant, and so on. The aim of Feng Shui is to create an environment where you can position yourself within harmonious chi.

Introducing the Concept of Feng Shui

Chi carries a constant flow of communication from the universe to Earth. Much chi stays around and within people, animals, plants, and buildings. Chi flows through you, around you, and out of you. This outward-flowing chi is a connecting and mixing chi. It connects you to another, the immediate environment, and at the same time, to the universe. This chi ripples to others and back from them like heat waves. These ripples carry much information in them, and it is this information a person who is psychic claims to understand. At the very least, it is from this ability to receive and understand these ripples of chi communication that we get our intuitive impressions and premonitions.

Of course it would have been out of character for the ancient Chinese to let these outer flows of chi just exist without making an attempt to harmonize with them. The chi energy that's taken into our bodies from our environment has a tremendous influence over our emotions and moods, our health and vital energy. We are also impacted by how chi flows through the environment.

Sensitive people can feel the emotional environment that's contained in any room or building. Others respond to it without understanding why their inner emotional environment has changed. A room where two people were just fighting will be highly charged, while a meditation room will be peaceful.

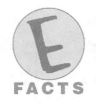

FACTS

I recently heard from a woman who was looking for a home to buy, and one stood out from all the rest. As soon as she walked in, she felt peaceful and was delighted with the floor layout. The difference from the other homes was so distinct that she wondered at it aloud. "Oh," the developer said, "I used a Feng Shui master in laying out the floor plan and in orienting the house. Do you like it?" Like it? She bought the house on the spot.

Chi is carried to Earth through the forces of nature—sunlight, wind, water, sound, and silence. It flows just as all of these do, with the exception of its permeability: It can flow through anything as well as around, over, under, and so on. It will flow more easily through some things than others. It flows well through natural fabrics and poorly through plastic. It flows easily around rounded corners, but sharp corners break up its flow. It is attracted to and has a nourishing relationship with plants, but becomes disorganized around TVs, computers, and microwaves. Chi is soothed by water and jumbled by intense traffic noise.

ESSENTIALS

The aim of Feng Shui is to create an environment where you can position yourself within harmonious chi. This chi carries within its very nature the qualities that are essential for you to relax, focus, and become your best self and realize your goals and your dreams. You can absorb these lovely flows into your own meridians and make their harmony yours.

The Chinese became adept at understanding the flow of chi and the qualities of chi that are essential to these realized life goals and dreams. If you don't understand how the chi flows, you can't understand how to best position yourself within it. The goal of the ancient Chinese architects and interior designers was to create buildings where chi could flow in harmony throughout. The interior design, then, enhanced these harmonious flows. This enhancing grew to such a precise art that inhabitants were interviewed as to their goals in life, their health and well-being, and concerns and problems. The interior was then "Feng Shui-ed" to create a chi environment in which these changes could be facilitated by the flowing chi.

Chi moves easily through doors, is more restricted by windows, and is reflected back by mirrors. This makes the orientation of the building to the sun and the planets important for determining the variety of chi entering the building. Other influencing factors are roads and bodies of water that are close by.

Improving Your Surroundings with Feng Shui

You can improve your own surroundings by employing simple Feng Shui techniques that get rid of the following bad types of chi. The idea behind Feng Shui-ing your T'ai Chi space is an exciting one. Don't feel that your building or home has to be well placed for Feng Shui to work. Any attempt to create a harmonious flow in any part of your home, even a small T'ai Chi space, is a worthy cause.

- **Negative chi:** Negative chi is chi that has been discombobulated by your use of synthetic building materials, artificial lighting, and air conditioning, so you want to limit or eliminate these unnatural surroundings.
- **Stagnant chi:** This is chi that is moving too slowly. This usually occurs in dark spaces and clutter, so move to lighten and clean spaces.
- **Fast-flowing chi:** This is chi that moves too quickly and is found in very long hallways and buildings with severe features.
- **Cutting chi:** This is when the natural flowing and rippling of the chi is cut by right angles. Feng Shui smoothes out sharp turns and softens corners.

Going Further with Feng Shui

You can find a number of good books on Feng Shui. After reading more, simply choose your space, follow the directions, and create a lovely spot in which to practice and feel the harmonious chi surrounding you.

One interesting aside is that cats love a Feng Shui-ed room. If you have a cat, he or she will probably make your practice space a favorite hangout!

CHAPTER 21

Continuing Your Practice

Now that you've gotten started with T'ai Chi and/or QiGong, you may need help in finding ways to continue practicing on a regular basis. This chapter will provide you with some tips.

Practicing T'ai Chi and QiGong Regularly Right from the Beginning

Be consistent in how much time you dedicate each day to each practice. Show up at about the same time each day. This practice of integrating QiGong and T'ai Chi into your life will create a body habit, and you'll be able to treat yourself to chi breaks and mini vacations at the drop of a hat. Use the calendars provided on pages 261–264 to keep track of your practice.

Body habits are powerful. Your lives are probably much more influenced by them than we realize. It is often a body habit that makes something feel right. It is a body habit that takes food and turns it into nurturing ourselves. It is body habit that allows muscles long unused to build up quickly when exercised years later. Your body's habits push you into action. We are looking to replace troubling body habits (overeating, excess shoulder tension, nervous habits) with useful body habits, habits that lend themselves to an improving inner and outer life.

It takes six weeks of steady commitment to form a body habit. This is because you're altering the nervous system. The nervous system thrives on variety. Creating a new body habit asks the nervous system to liven up its wiring by telling the muscles to do something a little different. The nervous system then helps memory store the movement into the muscle. This takes a while. Usually the older we get, the longer it may take to generate and complete this process. The nervous system of young people is quick to learn new things. The older we get, the more we live according to familiar habits and the more unchanging our body habits are. We move like we have always moved: Our mannerisms are the same. Over time, we change less and less in our body habits. We become programmed in our movements. In some ways, this is great because it creates predictable walking, sitting, stepping, and so on. The downside is that some muscles get overused and others are chronically underused. This creates movement stiffness and balance problems. The other problem is the nervous system isn't receiving what it loves—new, pleasant stimulation!

Being Consistent

Because the first six weeks are the hardest to make the time, be consistent. You have to make the effort to really do it, not just go through the motions. Life is so busy that you may be challenged to fit in one more activity, or you may lack sustained interest. Or, perhaps, a last minute change of plans keeps you from practicing. But if you continue to plod along taking T'ai Chi and QiGong space no matter what, time will begin to assist you. You will find that it gets easier and easier to have the time. Life will be more enjoyable, your health will improve, and a quiet state of mind will settle in.

ESSENTIALS

Through your practice, you will be more relaxed. Not couch-potato relaxed, but just truly relaxed, the way you'd like to feel all the time. When you commit to a regular practice session, you halt the buildup of tension your busy life creates in your muscles.

By doing the movements at a regular time (morning, midday, or evening) your body will develop the habit of putting down the built-up muscular tension. It is like setting down a heavy load you've been carrying all day and then letting your muscles rest. This relaxation settles into your body as you practice. Your mind slides into your movements. You have great relief from not thinking about the past, the future, or an imagined parallel present. The flowing breathing settles in. This occurs even if you know only a few positions. Put your whole self into them. Do what you know, repeat them in a flowing cycle. Settle down in the moment.

As you become consistent, your practice becomes a familiar body/mind memory for you. This memory strengthens over time from regular practice. A state of increasing relaxation creeps more and more into routine daily moments. You will find eventually that you're able to make a choice about how much tension you want to feel in any given event. Someone is rude, and you start to react, but a relaxed response has now become a part of your life. It is right there for you to draw from. You let the person's behavior roll right by you. You choose your own reaction. You're not controlled by stress responses that have built up over time. Life seems sweeter and happier. Your chi smoothes out and improves.

Time may also seem more spacious. In a world of multitasking and many activities drawing on you all at once, this sensation can feel like a miracle. Instead of the day feeling tightly wound around you, you have a feeling of spaciousness. Everyone else may still be feeling rushed, pressured, and harried. You, however, are feeling a bit more leisurely, a bit more confident that everything is in its right place. You may find that instead of running down a tunnel of stressed and focused thoughts, you now are aware of more of the world around you. It is the classic "take time to smell the roses."

Taking T'ai Chi and QiGong Breaks

One way to slow down is to take T'ai Chi and QiGong breaks wherever you are. Learning the movement and combining the breath and then engaging the mind are a perfect menu for refreshingly and stimulating R and R. The ongoing mastery of the breath and the movements call forth ever-increasing sensitivity that's required to continue to improve the movement. The type of sensitivity that T'ai Chi and QiGong call forth stimulates the nervous system, heightens it, and then feeds it with full and healthy chi. This, then, provides a wonderful combination for soothing stimulation. The art of having T'ai Chi and QiGong breaks becomes as natural as breathing.

You will find that simple snippets of QiGong or T'ai Chi occur to you during your day. While waiting in line somewhere you may find yourself shifting your weight slightly, moving the weight from being primarily on one leg and then the other. As you shift the weight, you will be experiencing T'ai Chi's full and empty, or yang and yin, teachings. As you gently shift the weight to one leg you can feel it fill, like a pitcher being filled with fluid, while your other leg is now empty and very light. Slowly, the weight can shift over. The full leg now loses its fullness to the empty leg. The previously empty leg is now full and deeply rooted in the ground. The line moves forward, and you move the empty leg first. You feel the firm rootedness of the full leg. You let the fullness pour into the empty leg that just changed position. This now full leg roots to the ground, and the newly empty leg moves forward. You can repeat this through the whole line.

Several great things have happened here. You've brought your busy, busy mind into the present. Your relaxed muscle memory of T'ai Chi has taken over the rest of your body. Your breath has deepened and become more normal. You've just spent five minutes in line and it has passed in a moment—a very constructive moment: a mini-vacation.

Or you may be sitting in a line of traffic. It may seem as if every person on the road is in collusion in trying to get in your way. You really need to relax and just let it be crowded, but how? The Reverse or Prebirth Breath mentioned in Chapter 5. It renews your energy level, focuses and calms your mind, brings the mind into being more present, and makes you more accepting of this inconvenience. I wouldn't recommend doing any form of QiGong or T'ai Chi when actually moving in your car, because it could distract you at a critical moment, so do your Prebirth Breath in the car only when you're stationary.

Driving does provide a perplexing problem. You may have to drive many hours a day, so being able to center and calm yourself while driving is of great value. What I suggest trying is a brief exercise before you enter the car. Form a habit or ritual. Before you get into your car, while you're actually walking toward it, relax your tan t'ien (see Chapter 1). Your belly will relax out a bit. Let a breath flow into you and then back out. Feel your shoulders relax down. Draw another breath and release it. Now imagine the air is breathing you. Your body is open and relaxed, and the air falls into you and now flows out. And now you're at your car, more centered and prepared for anything that comes your way.

Making a Commitment to an Expanded Life

Make a commitment to expand your awareness beyond your own self-contained life. We drive, phone, live up to responsibilities, make a living, get along with others, just to name a few. It is a lot, and it is all important, but not so important we can't expand our view of the moment to include more. A flower, a baby's smile, something funny, a great piece of music, a great memory are just a few gifts that await us if we include more in our self-lives.

FACTS

Using T'ai Chi methods of expanding awareness is an effective way to expand yourself to more pleasure in the ordinary moments. A relaxed person is naturally a more expanded person. A relaxed person appreciates more, enjoys giving more, receives with love, and sees more opportunities for him- or herself to enjoy still more.

If you become overwhelmed, use T'ai Chi to still your thoughts and expand your awareness. Are your kids driving you nuts at times, the noise, the busyness, the defiance—whatever? Put your fingers on your tan t'ien. Sink your breath to this point. Hold it for a second and exhale by releasing all the tension that is containing the inhale. Pull on your ears from top to lobes. Let your arms float up on an inhale, cross the arms over the chest, and put your hands around to the back of your neck. Take a literal step back and release your breath. Float your arms to your sides. You will feel more contained and ready to lay down boundaries that make sense for you and for them. Or you will be in a better position to turn tail and run to the nearest quiet space for a break!

APPENDIX A
Resources

Your model and teacher in this book, Fernando Raynolds, has instructional videos that can accompany this book. He also sends to his students newsletters with further instruction and information. To avail yourself of these, just drop him a letter at P.O. Box 1078, Talent, OR 97540; call him at 541-535-1778, or e-mail him at *dafrseb@wave.net*. Tell him what you need. He will either help you personally or refer you to another source.

Books

There are two books I love: *The Complete Book of T'ai Chi Ch'uan* by Wong Kiew Kit and *The Tao of T'ai Chi Ch'uan Way to Rejuvenation* by Jou Tsung Hwa. These are written by two skilled T'ai Chi Ch'uan masters. Jou Tsung Hwa passed away a few years ago; he had a dream of a T'ai Chi Ch'uan university, and his book was a textbook he wrote should such a school develop. Both books are excellent, precise, and complete.

Magazines and Videos

Check out *T'ai Chi Magazine* at ✒ *www.tai-chi.com* (on the Internet) or ⊞ P.O. Box 39938, Los Angeles, CA 90039 (via mail). Remember, the form taught in this magazine is Yang Style, so in seeking further guidance, be clear on the form.

T'ai Chi Magazine has advertisements about instruction camps in beautiful places. Call them at ☎ 800-888-9119, or send an e-mail to ✒ *taichi@tai-chi.com*.

T'ai Chi Music & Videos
✒ *www.sportsmusic.com/chi.html*

SMI Music and Videos
✒ *www.taichivideostore.com*

Ron Perfetti Instructional Videos
✒ *www.maui.net/~taichi4u/taichi.html*

Qigong Videos
✒ *www.sal4healing.com*

The Internet

The Internet is full of T'ai Chi and QiGong Web sites. Some are filled with free information, while others are ads for products. T'ai Chi and

QiGong practitioners are a group of enthusiastic people. Make contact through chat rooms or e-mail, and you will find you've entered a network of helpful and obliging people.

T'ai Chi

Yang Family T'ai Chi Ch'uan Site
www.yangfamilytaichi.com

Xiong Jing School of T'ai Chi Ch'uan
www.xiongjing.com

Chen-style T'ai Chi Ch'uan
www.chentaichi.com

Wu Style Jai Ji Quan Form
www.wfdesign.com/tc

Easy T'ai Chi for Busy People
www.easytaichi.com

T'ai Chi Academy, Sunnyvale, California
www.taichiacademy.com

The T'ai Chi Site: News, Links, Discussions
www.thetaichisite.com

T'ai Chi Productions
www.taichiproduction.com

Tantra T'ai Chi
www.tantrataichi.com

Golden T'ai Chi for Seniors
www.taichiforseniors.com

T'ai Chi for Older People
www.nih.gov/nia/new/press/taichi.htm

T'ai Chi links
http://scheele.org/lee/tcclinks.html

QiGong

National Qigong Association of America
www.nqa.org

American Qigong Association
www.eastwestqi.com/aqa

History of Qigong
www.acupuncture.com/qikung/history.htm

Message Boards

www.mtsu.edu/~jpurcell/taichi/taichi
www.gates.com/bbs-tai/tai-chi1.html

Shopping

Gaiam: A Lifestyle Company
www.gaiam.com

Travel

Lake Austin Spa Resort
www.lakeaustin.com

The Heartland Health Spa
www.heartland/spa.com/activities.11

Month

SUNDAY	MONDAY	TUESDAY	WEDNESDAY	THURSDAY	FRIDAY	SATURDAY

Month _____

SUNDAY	MONDAY	TUESDAY	WEDNESDAY	THURSDAY	FRIDAY	SATURDAY

Month _____

SUNDAY	MONDAY	TUESDAY	WEDNESDAY	THURSDAY	FRIDAY	SATURDAY

Month _____

SUNDAY	MONDAY	TUESDAY	WEDNESDAY	THURSDAY	FRIDAY	SATURDAY

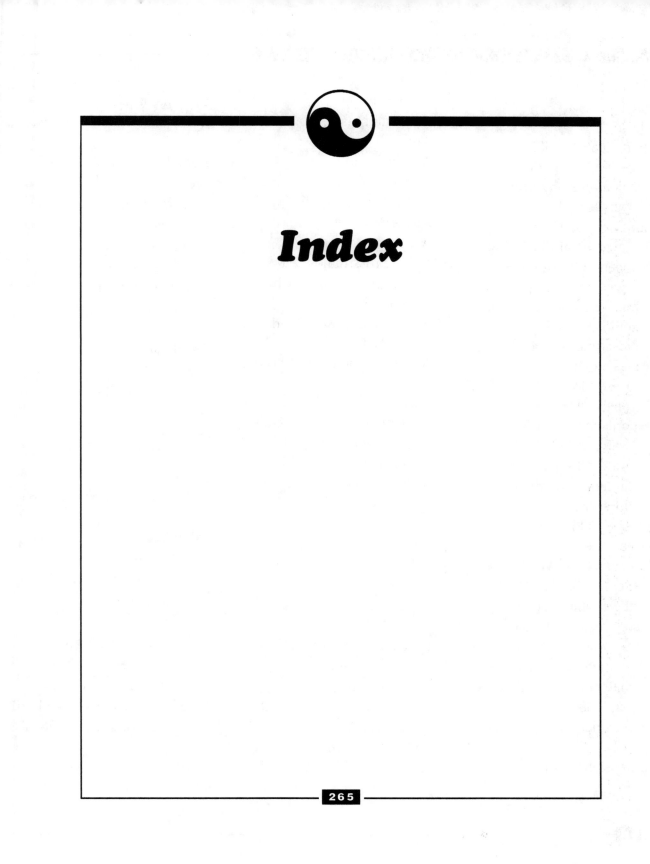

Index

We Have EVERYTHING!

Everything® **After College Book**
$12.95, 1-55850-847-3

Everything® **American History Book**
$12.95, 1-58062-531-2

Everything® **Angels Book**
$12.95, 1-58062-398-0

Everything® **Anti-Aging Book**
$12.95, 1-58062-565-7

Everything® **Astrology Book**
$12.95, 1-58062-062-0

Everything® **Baby Names Book**
$12.95, 1-55850-655-1

Everything® **Baby Shower Book**
$12.95, 1-58062-305-0

Everything® **Baby's First Food Book**
$12.95, 1-58062-512-6

Everything® **Baby's First Year Book**
$12.95, 1-58062-581-9

Everything® **Barbeque Cookbook**
$12.95, 1-58062-316-6

Everything® **Bartender's Book**
$9.95, 1-55850-536-9

Everything® **Bedtime Story Book**
$12.95, 1-58062-147-3

Everything® **Bicycle Book**
$12.00, 1-55850-706-X

Everything® **Breastfeeding Book**
$12.95, 1-58062-582-7

Everything® **Build Your Own Home Page**
$12.95, 1-58062-339-5

Everything® **Business Planning Book**
$12.95, 1-58062-491-X

Everything® **Candlemaking Book**
$12.95, 1-58062-623-8

Everything® **Casino Gambling Book**
$12.95, 1-55850-762-0

Everything® **Cat Book**
$12.95, 1-55850-710-8

Everything® **Chocolate Cookbook**
$12.95, 1-58062-405-7

Everything® **Christmas Book**
$15.00, 1-55850-697-7

Everything® **Civil War Book**
$12.95, 1-58062-366-2

Everything® **Classical Mythology Book**
$12.95, 1-58062-653-X

Everything® **Collectibles Book**
$12.95, 1-58062-645-9

Everything® **College Survival Book**
$12.95, 1-55850-720-5

Everything® **Computer Book**
$12.95, 1-58062-401-4

Everything® **Cookbook**
$14.95, 1-58062-400-6

Everything® **Cover Letter Book**
$12.95, 1-58062-312-3

Everything® **Creative Writing Book**
$12.95, 1-58062-647-5

Everything® **Crossword and Puzzle Book**
$12.95, 1-55850-764-7

Everything® **Dating Book**
$12.95, 1-58062-185-6

Everything® **Dessert Book**
$12.95, 1-55850-717-5

Everything® **Digital Photography Book**
$12.95, 1-58062-574-6

Everything® **Dog Book**
$12.95, 1-58062-144-9

Everything® **Dreams Book**
$12.95, 1-55850-806-6

Everything® **Etiquette Book**
$12.95, 1-55850-807-4

Everything® **Fairy Tales Book**
$12.95, 1-58062-546-0

Everything® **Family Tree Book**
$12.95, 1-55850-763-9

Everything® **Feng Shui Book**
$12.95, 1-58062-587-8

Everything® **Fly-Fishing Book**
$12.95, 1-58062-148-1

Everything® **Games Book**
$12.95, 1-55850-643-8

Everything® **Get-A-Job Book**
$12.95, 1-58062-223-2

Everything® **Get Out of Debt Book**
$12.95, 1-58062-588-6

Everything® **Get Published Book**
$12.95, 1-58062-315-8

Everything® **Get Ready for Baby Book**
$12.95, 1-55850-844-9

Everything® **Get Rich Book**
$12.95, 1-58062-670-X

Everything® **Ghost Book**
$12.95, 1-58062-533-9

Everything® **Golf Book**
$12.95, 1-55850-814-7

Everything® **Grammar and Style Book**
$12.95, 1-58062-573-8

Everything® **Guide to Las Vegas**
$12.95, 1-58062-438-3

Everything® **Guide to New England**
$12.95, 1-58062-589-4

Everything® **Guide to New York City**
$12.95, 1-58062-314-X

Everything® **Guide to Walt Disney World®,
Universal Studios®, and
Greater Orlando, 2nd Edition**
$12.95, 1-58062-404-9

Everything® **Guide to Washington D.C.**
$12.95, 1-58062-313-1

Everything® **Guitar Book**
$12.95, 1-58062-555-X

Everything® **Herbal Remedies Book**
$12.95, 1-58062-331-X

Available wherever books are sold!
To order, call 800-872-5627, or visit everything.com
Adams Media Corporation, 57 Littlefield Street, Avon, MA 02322. U.S.A.

Everything® **Home-Based Business Book**
$12.95, 1-58062-364-6

Everything® **Homebuying Book**
$12.95, 1-58062-074-4

Everything® **Homeselling Book**
$12.95, 1-58062-304-2

Everything® **Horse Book**
$12.95, 1-58062-564-9

Everything® **Hot Careers Book**
$12.95, 1-58062-486-3

Everything® **Internet Book**
$12.95, 1-58062-073-6

Everything® **Investing Book**
$12.95, 1-58062-149-X

Everything® **Jewish Wedding Book**
$12.95, 1-55850-801-5

Everything® **Job Interview Book**
$12.95, 1-58062-493-6

Everything® **Lawn Care Book**
$12.95, 1-58062-487-1

Everything® **Leadership Book**
$12.95, 1-58062-513-4

Everything® **Learning French Book**
$12.95, 1-58062-649-1

Everything® **Learning Spanish Book**
$12.95, 1-58062-575-4

Everything® **Low-Fat High-Flavor
Cookbook**
$12.95, 1-55850-802-3

Everything® **Magic Book**
$12.95, 1-58062-418-9

Everything® **Managing People Book**
$12.95, 1-58062-577-0

Everything® **Microsoft® Word 2000 Book**
$12.95, 1-58062-306-9

Everything® **Money Book**
$12.95, 1-58062-145-7

Everything® **Mother Goose Book**
$12.95, 1-58062-490-1

Everything® **Motorcycle Book**
$12.95, 1-58062-554-1

Everything® **Mutual Funds Book**
$12.95, 1-58062-419-7

Everything® **One-Pot Cookbook**
$12.95, 1-58062-186-4

Everything® **Online Business Book**
$12.95, 1-58062-320-4

Everything® **Online Genealogy Book**
$12.95, 1-58062-402-2

Everything® **Online Investing Book**
$12.95, 1-58062-338-7

Everything® **Online Job Search Book**
$12.95, 1-58062-365-4

Everything® **Organize Your Home Book**
$12.95, 1-58062-617-3

Everything® **Pasta Book**
$12.95, 1-55850-719-1

Everything® **Philosophy Book**
$12.95, 1-58062-644-0

Everything® **Playing Piano and
Keyboards Book**
$12.95, 1-58062-651-3

Everything® **Pregnancy Book**
$12.95, 1-58062-146-5

Everything® **Pregnancy Organizer**
$15.00, 1-58062-336-0

Everything® **Project Management Book**
$12.95, 1-58062-583-5

Everything® **Puppy Book**
$12.95, 1-58062-576-2

Everything® **Quick Meals Cookbook**
$12.95, 1-58062-488-X

Everything® **Resume Book**
$12.95, 1-58062-311-5

Everything® **Romance Book**
$12.95, 1-58062-566-5

Everything® **Running Book**
$12.95, 1-58062-618-1

Everything® **Sailing Book, 2nd Edition**
$12.95, 1-58062-671-8

Everything® **Saints Book**
$12.95, 1-58062-534-7

Everything® **Selling Book**
$12.95, 1-58062-319-0

Everything® **Shakespeare Book**
$12.95, 1-58062-591-6

Everything® **Spells and Charms Book**
$12.95, 1-58062-532-0

Everything® **Start Your Own Business Book**
$12.95, 1-58062-650-5

Everything® **Stress Management Book**
$12.95, 1-58062-578-9

Everything® **Study Book**
$12.95, 1-55850-615-2

Everything® **Tai Chi and QiGong Book**
$12.95, 1-58062-646-7

Everything® **Tall Tales, Legends, and
Outrageous Lies Book**
$12.95, 1-58062-514-2

Everything® **Tarot Book**
$12.95, 1-58062-191-0

Everything® **Time Management Book**
$12.95, 1-58062-492-8

Everything® **Toasts Book**
$12.95, 1-58062-189-9

Everything® **Toddler Book**
$12.95, 1-58062-592-4

Everything® **Total Fitness Book**
$12.95, 1-58062-318-2

Everything® **Trivia Book**
$12.95, 1-58062-143-0

Everything® **Tropical Fish Book**
$12.95, 1-58062-343-3

Everything® **Vegetarian Cookbook**
$12.95, 1-58062-640-8

Everything® **Vitamins, Minerals,
and Nutritional
Supplements Book**
$12.95, 1-58062-496-0

Everything® **Wedding Book, 2nd Edition**
$12.95, 1-58062-190-2

Everything® **Wedding Checklist**
$7.95, 1-58062-456-1

Everything® **Wedding Etiquette Book**
$7.95, 1-58062-454-5

Everything® **Wedding Organizer**
$15.00, 1-55850-828-7

Everything® **Wedding Shower Book**
$7.95, 1-58062-188-0

Everything® **Wedding Vows Book**
$7.95, 1-58062-455-3

Everything® **Weight Training Book**
$12.95, 1-58062-593-2

Everything® **Wine Book**
$12.95, 1-55850-808-2

Everything® **World War II Book**
$12.95, 1-58062-572-X

Everything® **World's Religions Book**
$12.95, 1-58062-648-3

Everything® **Yoga Book**
$12.95, 1-58062-594-0

Visit us at everything.com

Everything® is a registered trademark of Adams Media Corporation.

OTHER *EVERYTHING*® BOOKS BY ADAMS MEDIA CORPORATION

EVERYTHING®

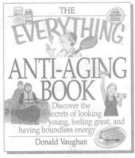

Trade Paperback, $12.95
1-58062-578-9, 304 pages

The Everything® Stress Management Book
Eve Adamson

The Everything® *Stress Management Book* provides the most effective methods of stress reduction and helpful hints on how to prevent stress from building up before it leads to chronic health problems. It explains the latest, most potent techniques for quelling anxiety, including simple exercises, stress-fighting foods, aromatherapy, yoga, and massage. Full of charts, tables, important warnings, and useful tips, *The Everything*® *Stress Management Book* is a complete guide on how to achieve life's goals—without wearing down the human body.

The Everything® Anti-Aging Book
Donald Vaughan

Trade Paperback, $12.95
1-58062-565-7, 304 pages

Containing the most up-to-date anti-aging research available, *The Everything*® *Anti-Aging Book* is the essential resource for both the young in body and the young at heart. It explains the aging process in simple terms, and details the many methods of slowing down natural aging to improve physical and mental health and quality of life. Packed with tips on everything from nutrition and exercise to spirituality and herbal remedies, this easy-to-follow reference teaches you how to age healthfully and gracefully.

Available wherever books are sold!
To order, call 800-872-5627, or visit everything.com
Adams Media Corporation, 57 Littlefield Street, Avon, MA 02322. U.S.A.